MINDFUL MUSLIMAH

A Muslim Woman's Guide to Meditation and Spirituality

M. Hasen

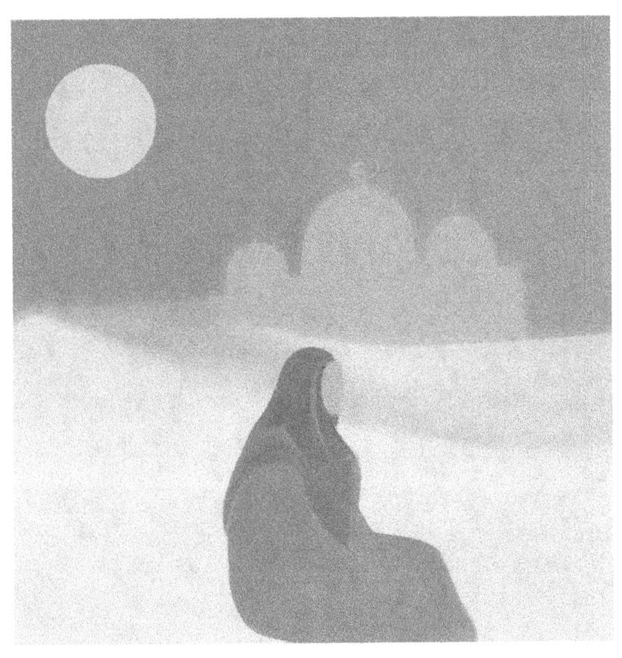

DEDICATED

*To **Mother***

CONTENTS

Title Page   1

Dedicated   3

About this book   6

Introduction   8

Slow down   12

brings comfort to your heart   16

Cleaning Meditation: Transforming Chores into a Mindful Practice   20

three Minutes Meditation   23

Small deeds, Big rewards: The Power of Daily Progress   27

5 Minutes challenge to get things done   32

Small Habits, Big Streams of Rewards   34

what really matters to you?   50

How Knowing Your Worth Can Change Your Life?   56

conserve your brain energy   59

Simplicity and Happiness: How Less Can Truly Be More   62

Balance Between Ambition and Gratitude   70

Gratitude   74

Positive thinking 76

can money truly buy happiness? 79

The Freedom of Forgiveness: Release Your Burdens 82

Overcoming Laziness: Islamic Perspectives 87

The Importance of Real Socializing: Why Technology 97
Can't Replace Human Connection

Beliefs and Behaviors:The Power of Positive Self- 102
Image

The Myth of Multitasking: How It Can Actually Slow 106
You Down

110

Avoid Digital Distractions : Take Control of Your Foucs

115

Read Your Way to Riches

Don't buy a yoga mat : Finding Peace on the Prayer 118
Mat

Connect with us 121

ABOUT THIS **BOOK**

"Those who believe, and whose hearts find satisfaction in the remembrance of Allah: for without doubt in the remembrance of Allah do hearts find satisfaction." - Quran 13:28

"Islamic meditation" differs from contemporary meditation in that it is centered around the remembrance of Allah and living a pious and God-fearing life, rather than sitting on a yoga mat and chanting mantras or calling spirits into the room. The goal of **"Islamic meditation"** is to attain inner **peace** and **happiness** by pleasing Allah and showing mercy towards humanity, with the ultimate aim of attaining the rewards of the hereafter. You can't truly be at **peace** or happy until your God is happy with you and you've put your trust in Him.

While there is no such term in Islam, I will be using "Mediation" to refer to the practices in Islam that serve the same purposes as contemporary meditation and mindfulness.

In today's world, where stress and anxiety are widespread, mindfulness and spiritual reflection are essential. The purpose of mindfulness is to cultivate self-awareness, inner **peace**, and clarity of thought, all of which can be attained through the teachings of Islam. This book aims to provide women with an easy-to-follow guide on how to incorporate Islamic meditation into their daily routines, taking into account the unique needs and responsibilities of women.

This book is a concise read, and it doesn't elaborate on everything. Rather, it leaves many aspects open for the reader to interpret and draw meaning from. As you read through the book, you will encounter words like **peace, happiness, kindness, compassion, focus, and spirituality**. These are all crucial aspects of meditation, and by incorporating Islamic teachings and practices into your life, you can achieve them.

*May Allah guide us all towards a fulfilling and **peaceful** life. Ameen.*

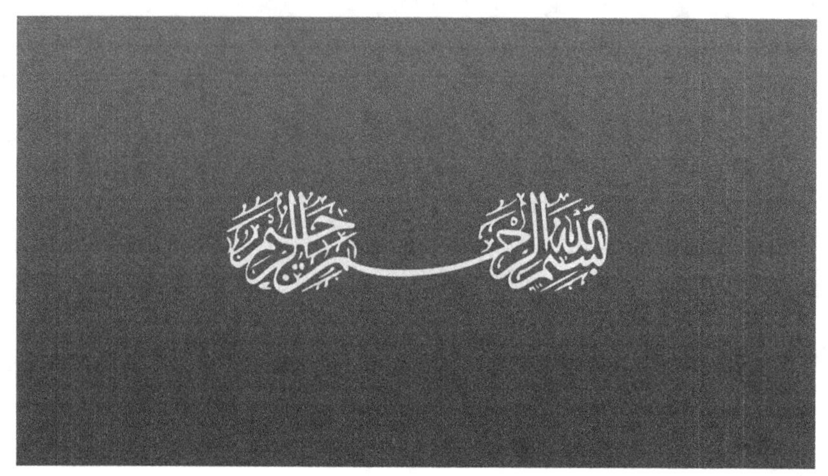

INTRODUCTION

Have you ever thought about meditating but felt like you needed a yoga mat, a quiet space, and an instructor to guide you through it? Well, guess what? That's not true! You don't need any of those things to start meditating.

Let's try it together. Take a deep breath and exhale slowly. Congratulations! You just meditated! How do you feel? Present in the moment, right?

Meditation is a great way to reduce stress and anxiety, and you can do it anytime, anywhere. You don't need a yoga mat or a special place. In fact, you can even do it while driving or waiting for your *five-time salah* (Muslim Prayer). This book comes with a *virtual* yoga mat that you can use whenever and wherever you want - whether you're walking, cooking, dusting, traveling, commuting, lying in bed, or just taking a break. So, let's get started on our meditation journey together.

Have you ever wondered why we don't meditate more often? It seems like we're always making excuses or finding reasons not to do it. We create mental barriers and convince ourselves that we're not ready or that we need certain things in order to start meditating. Our motivation to meditate might last for a few days or even a few weeks, but eventually, we find ourselves making excuses and procrastinating. It's like we're stabbing our own enthusiasm with the dagger of excuses.

Think about your daily routine. It's a constant rush to get everything done - getting ready, making breakfast, taking care of the kids, and then rushing off to work or school. We face all kinds of pressures and stresses throughout the day, and by the time we get home, we're exhausted. And what do we do to unwind? We turn on the TV or scroll through social media - which can actually make us feel even more anxious or depressed. It's a vicious cycle, and before we know it, another day has passed us by.

I'm not going to tell you to hit the gym after a long day or hush your kids to find a quiet spot in your house to lay down a yoga mat. Sure, these things are great, like spending an hour at the gym, jogging for 30 minutes every day, meditating, drinking no sugar coffee, green tea, and a glass of water on an empty stomach. But let's be honest, you've probably tried all of these things before, only to lose steam and fall back into your old habits. That's why I'm here to tell you that it's okay, and it's actually easier than you might think to start and maintain these healthy habits. All you need to do is read this book with an open mind, and I promise you'll see a real difference in your life.

By reading this book and taking its advice, you can make tiny changes that will have a big impact on your overall wellbeing. For example, moving the Quran to a more prominent place in your home, taking deep breaths throughout the day, or relocating your smartphone app icons can all make a difference. Even disabling fingerprint unlocking and changing your mobile password can be small but important steps towards a healthier lifestyle. Let this book be your guide to making lasting, positive changes in your life.

Reeelaaax and Read slowly. (*good. you are taking a deep breath*). Don't rush through the text, as you will gain more enjoyment by taking your time. I suggest reading one chapter per day, allowing yourself a full day to absorb the message and implement the suggestions before moving on to the next chapter.

[Take the first step]
You'll notice this sign all throughout the book. When you see it, make a promise to give it a try. Trust me, you'll notice an instant change in yourself. Insha'Allah!

The goal of this book is to help you achieve the benefits

of meditation without actually breathing in and breathing out on a yoga mat. While you might not discover anything totally new here, my aim is to draw your attention to the small details we often overlook in our everyday lives. By doing so, I hope to assist you in creating powerful habits that will improve your mental, emotional, and spiritual wellbeing. I'll be keeping it brief and straightforward, and you might notice that I repeat myself at times to drive a point home.

Ready? Imagine spreading out your virtual yoga mat and take a **Deeeeep Breath** *in.*

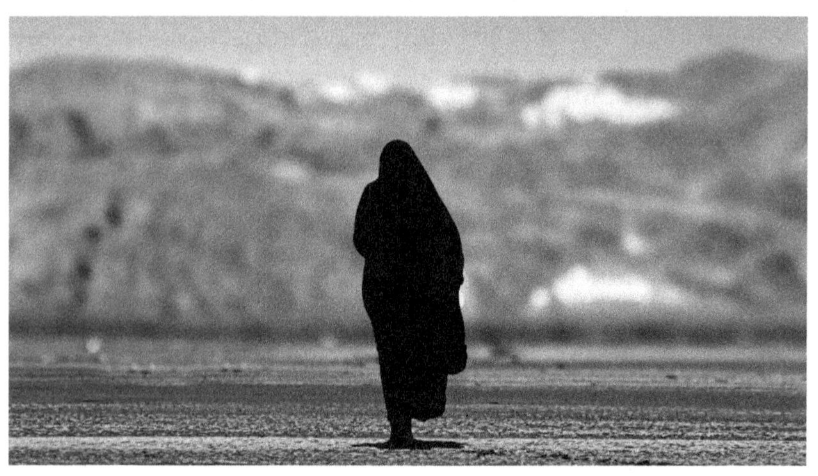

SLOW DOWN

Do you ever feel like there just aren't enough hours in the day to get everything done? It seems like we're always expected to do more and more, and we put so much pressure on ourselves to be constantly productive. But when we don't accomplish everything we set out to do, it can lead to feelings of anxiety and frustration.

Have you noticed that we're always rushing around, trying to finish one task after another? Even when we're praying, our minds can be preoccupied with all the things we have to do next. It can be hard to slow down, but it's so important for our mental health.

So here's a suggestion: take a deep breath and *slooow down* a bit (Good you took a deep breath). Whenever you feel like you're getting overwhelmed, just pause for a moment and let yourself relax. Slowing down can actually be a great way to combat anxiety and stress.

So why not give it a try?

Yes, that's it. Read it slow.

If you slow down while walking around your office or doing your daily household chores, your breath will naturally slow down and your body will start to relax? When you're more relaxed, you'll feel less stressed and more in control of your day. So why not take a few deep breaths and try slowing down your pace next time you're going about your day? Your body and mind will thank you for it!

[Take the first step]

*Go and grab a glass of water and when you head to the kitchen walk **slooowly***

Have you ever noticed how we can form opinions about someone just by the way they walk? It's because our walk is associated with our behavior, level of control, confidence, and attitude. And get this, just by changing the way we walk, we can actually affect the way we think and behave. It might sound crazy, but try it out and see for yourself - when you walk differently, you'll notice a change in your attitude too.

Another thing to try out is walking slowly or taking slow, deliberate steps. It's almost like a form of meditation, similar to the Chinese practice of Tai Chi. As you move through each step, focus on your breathing and stay present in the moment. Not only is it good exercise, but it can also help clear your mind and reduce stress.

I can tell that you're already feeling the effects - you know it's really working!

So whenever you think you are stressing out, in the office or at home, whatever you are doing just *S L O W   D O W N*. I promise you will notice an instant change in yourself. This will also help you in increasing focus. You will find a boring task a little less boring. I know what you are thinking. You can't enjoy dusting or doing the dishes and nothing can make it enjoyable.

So whenever you feel like you're getting stressed out - whether it's at work or at home - just remember to slow down. I guarantee you'll notice an instant change in yourself. It will also help you increase your focus, You will find a boring task a little less boring.

I know what you might be thinking - there's no way to make doing something like dusting or doing the dishes enjoyable. But here's the thing: When you slow down and really give your full attention to whatever you're doing, you're actually meditating! It's all about shifting your mindset and approaching the task with a new perspective.

So next time you're feeling super stressed or overwhelmed, try slowing down and taking your time with whatever it is you need to do. Just take it step by step, and don't rush to finish it. Instead, take the time to really observe yourself doing it. If it doesn't work for you, you can always go back to your old ways. But it's worth a shot, right?

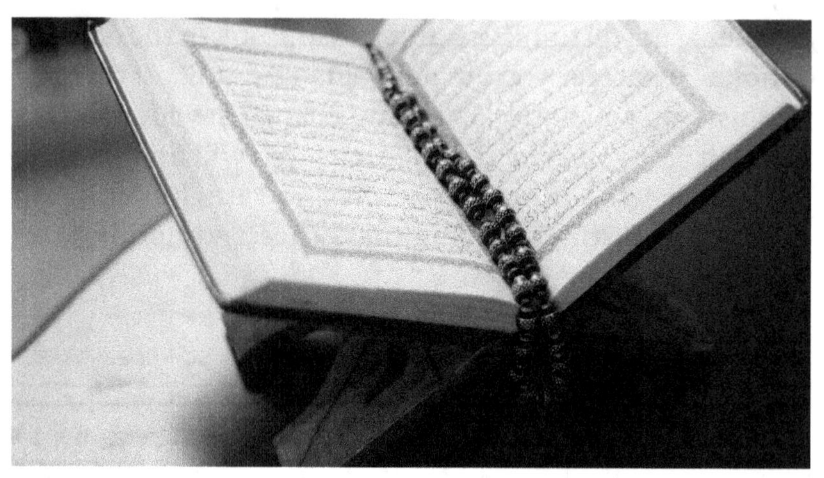

BRINGS COMFORT
TO YOUR **HEART**

Our minds are powerful tools, but we need to learn to control them. Our thoughts can affect our focus, concentration, stress levels, **happiness**, and even our mental and physical health. While meditation is hard to define, there are some common goals that people aim to achieve through this practice. Firstly, meditation can help to reduce stress, anxiety, depression, and pain. It's a way to find **peace** amidst life's chaos. Secondly, it can increase our attention and awareness, helping us to be more present in the moment. Finally, meditation can help us achieve a mentally clear, emotionally calm state.

Meditation is a practice that's embraced by people all

around the world. Many different cultures have their own forms of traditional meditation, including the Hindu, Buddhist, and Sufi traditions. For example, chanting meditation - like the Hindu chant "uhm" - can be used to distract oneself from the outside world. But there are other types of meditation as well. One approach involves focusing your attention intently on one specific thing, like your breathing. The idea is to keep your focus strongly fixed on that one point, and continuously bring your attention back to it whenever your mind starts to wander. Another approach is to simply pay attention to everything that's happening around you without reacting to it. It's all about noticing and being present in the moment.

There are many potential benefits of meditation that are still being researched and discovered. From improved mental and physical health to increased overall well-being, there's a lot to explore and gain through this powerful practice.

Mindfulness

When it comes to mindfulness meditation, it's all about simplicity and effectiveness. All you need to do is sit upright and focus on your breath. The goal is to stay present in the moment and let go of distractions, like daydreaming or worrying about the past and future. However, the real exercise comes from redirecting your attention back to your breath when your mind starts to wander. It can be challenging at first, but with practice, you'll gradually increase your focus time and improve your ability to stay present. By challenging lifelong habits of daydreaming, remorse, or fear, you can break the cycle of thoughts that constantly occupy your mind, even during sleep. When your thoughts drift away, gently bring them back to the present moment and continue to practice.

Control Your Mind's Thoughts Instead Of Your Mind Controls You.

Research shows that eight weeks of mediation can change your brain size. This can lead to greater capacity for learning, improved focus, decreased fear, stress, anxiety, and better control over bad habits and blood pressure. Meditation can be done in a variety of positions, such as sitting, lying down, standing, or even while working. The key is to maintain focus on your desired result. You can even incorporate activities that already bring you a sense of calm and mindfulness, such as **Salah,** reading **Quran, Dhikr (zikr), or charity.**

Allah said in the Quran, "Those who believe, and whose hearts find comfort in the remembrance of Allah. Surely, it is in the remembrance of Allah that hearts find comfort" (Quran 13:28).

*Incorporating meditation into your life through these practices can help bring about a greater sense of **peace** and comfort in your daily life.*

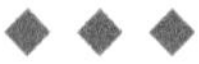

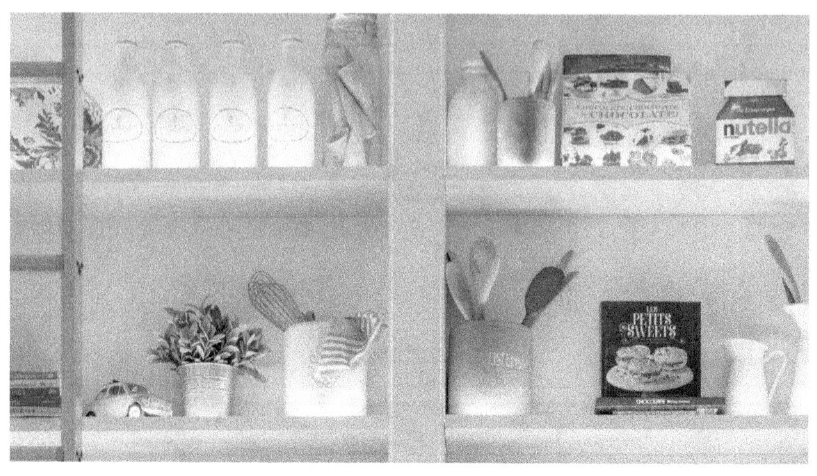

CLEANING MEDITATION: TRANSFORMING CHORES INTO A MINDFUL PRACTICE

"Cleanliness is half of faith (iman) " Prophet Muhammad (peace be upon him)

Have you ever noticed how your surroundings can affect your mental state? It's true! For example, when you're trying to pray in a cluttered and messy space, it's easy for your mind to get distracted by the untidiness around you. As they say, "a cluttered desk is a cluttered mind. **Think about it - when you walk into someone's home and it's messy and dirty, how does that make you feel? It's hard to focus on anything else but the mess!**

On the other hand, imagine walking into a room with perfect lighting and just a simple writing table and chair in the corner. How would that make you feel? Your surroundings can set the mood and mode for your mindset.

[Take the first step]

TAKE A PICTURE OF YOUR ROOM OR KITCHEN BEFORE AND AFTER YOU TIDY UP? IT'S A GREAT WAY TO SEE THE PROGRESS YOU'VE MADE AND FEEL GOOD ABOUT THE RESULTS. JUST IMAGINE, YOU CAN LOOK AT THE PICTURES SIDE BY SIDE AND SEE THE DIFFERENCE. HOW DOES IT MAKE YOU FEEL? TRY IT OUT AND SEE FOR YOURSELF!

Cleaning and organizing your home is more about creativity than spending money. If you change your attitude towards it, you can view it as a form of self-expression. After all, everyone has different tastes and preferences, which is why no two homes look exactly the same. You can use your own aesthetic sense to choose colors, textures, and lighting that appeal to you.

Have you ever watched those videos where people use tons of creativity to organize their homes? They call it an art or a craft! If you're in need of inspiration, check out minimalist home interiors or videos on the art of organizing a home. Who knows, you might even discover a new passion!

You might not think of cleaning as a form of meditation, but believe it or not, it can be! Even if you hate doing dishes or dusting, you can still incorporate mindfulness into your cleaning routine. ***There's a saying from the Prophet Muhammad (peace be upon him) that goes, "Cleanliness is half of faith"***. Not only is cleaning your space good for your physical health, but it can also be good for your spiritual health.

Here are three simple steps you can follow to turn cleaning into a meditative experience:
-Take a deep breath
-Go slow
-Observe yourself doing

Walla! You are meditating

You've officially turned your cleaning time into a moment of mindfulness. Take a moment to admire the clean environment, give yourself a compliment, and even smile. You'll be much happier in a clean and clutter-free space. So, from now on, don't think of cleaning as a chore
*- **treat it like an art form and become an artist of your own space today!***

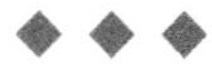

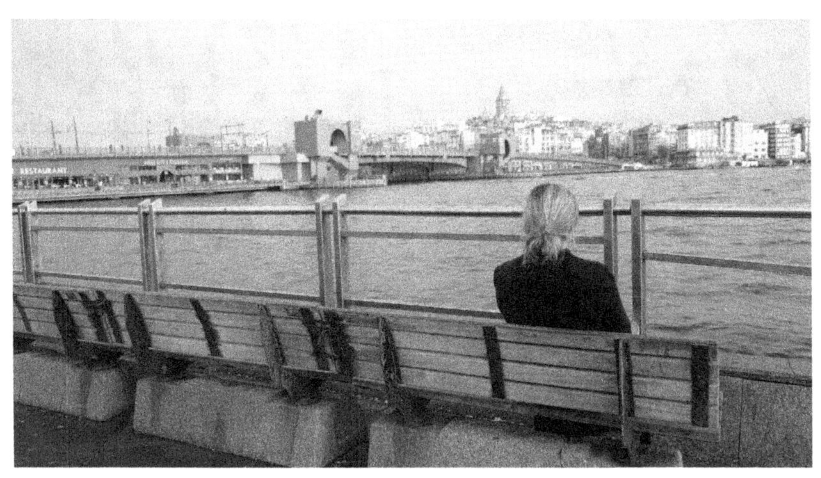

THREE MINUTES
MEDITATION

Find three minutes every day to sit and do NOTHING. Yes, nothing.

Find just three minutes each day to sit and do absolutely nothing? **Yes, you read that right** - nothing! I know it may sound impossible at first, but give it a try for a few days. While I personally believe that meditation should come naturally rather than being a deliberate effort, taking that initial step can help make it a habit. And trust me, after just a few days, you'll start to find it interesting and beneficial. I promise that if you stick to it, you'll thank me for the rest of your life. *So why not give it a go?*

Make three minutes for yourself. Find a quiet spot, sit with your legs apart, and let your palms rest at your sides. Take a deep breath and try to clear your mind. I know, it's not easy to stop thinking, but with practice, it will get better. The key is to monitor your thoughts and notice when your mind drifts away from the present moment. Once you notice this happening, gently guide your thoughts back to the here and now. Trust me, with time and practice, you'll become better at it.

When you're taking those three minutes for yourself, remind yourself that this time is just for relaxation. It's like you're taking a mini-vacation from your worries, plans, and responsibilities. Make the most out of these few minutes and let yourself unwind.

Here's a tip for better memorization and increased creativity. Whenever you're studying or trying to remember something, take a break for just three minutes. Don't touch your phone, instead take a deeeep breath and sit quietly. Let your brain absorb what you've learned so far. It works wonders! You can also do it after finishing a task before moving to the next one. Just sit back and do nothing. It helps you relax and feel less stressed. If you're a creative person, taking a three-minute break for meditation can help you come up with new and innovative ideas. Sometimes we get stuck in a problem and keep trying the same thing over and over again. Taking a short break can give you fresh waves of ideas and different angles to think from.

For the best results, move away from your workplace and enjoy the benefits of a three-minute meditation break.

Did you know that you can even meditate while doing your daily chores? Yeh! It's true! Whether you're dusting, cleaning, or doing the dishes, just take 3 minutes to slow down and focus on the present moment. And guess what? You can even meditate while driving! No need to pull over, just switch to the slower lane and take 3 minutes to relax and focus on your breath. Not only will you feel more alert and aware of your surroundings, but you'll also notice your shoulders relaxing and your breathing deepening. You might even start noticing things in your surroundings that you don't usually pay attention to throughout the day. Give it a try and see how it works for you!

[*Take the first step]*

PUT THIS BOOK DOWN, TAKE A DEEP BREATH, SIT QUIETLY AND TRY NOT TO THINK ABOUT ANYTHING. JUST ALLOW YOURSELF TO BE STILL AND PRESENT IN THE MOMENT.

Remember, everything can wait for just three minutes. It may seem like a long time at first, especially during that first minute when it's most difficult to quiet your mind. You may feel an itch, a craving for a snack, or the temptation to check your phone. But when you notice these distractions, just gently bring your mind back to the present moment and let them go. With practice, you'll find it easier to sit still and be present without feeling the urge to do something else.

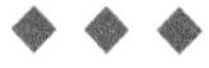

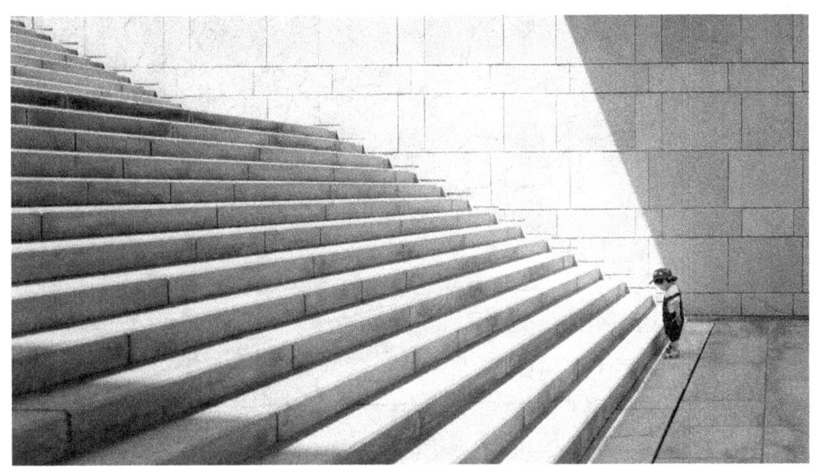

SMALL DEEDS, BIG REWARDS: THE POWER OF **DAILY** PROGRESS

Starting a new goal is always so exciting, isn't it? We feel energetic, motivated, and ready to take on the world. But then, as we start working on our goal, we begin to focus on how far we are from reaching it, and that can be discouraging. We might even start procrastinating and leaving things incomplete, feeling frustrated that we're not making enough progress. The thing is, when we're too focused on the end goal, we can lose sight of the progress we've already made, and that can sap our energy and excitement.

Have you heard of the Japanese technique called **"kaizen"**? It's all about the philosophy of constant progress and the development of good habits. It reminds me of a Hadith of prophet muhammad (Peace be upon him) -

"Take on only as much as you can do of good deeds, for the best of deeds is that which is done consistently, even if it is little." (Sunan Ibn Majah, Book of Zuhd, Hadith 4240)

This philosophy is perfect for anyone who wants to make steady progress towards their goals. Instead of overwhelming ourselves with too much, we can focus on consistent, gradual improvement.

The beauty of the kaizen philosophy is that it encourages you to take small steps towards your goals consistently over time. It's like working out at the gym - you can't expect to see immediate results, but with regular effort, you will start to notice changes over time. This can be incredibly helpful if you're feeling stuck, frustrated, or like giving up on your goals. Instead of trying to make huge changes all at once, focus on taking small steps towards your goal every day. This consistent effort will eventually lead to big results, and you'll be amazed at how far you've come.

Keep reminding yourself of this Hadith whenever you feel like giving up due to slow progress. Remember that progress takes time, and consistency is key. Don't get discouraged by slow progress, instead focus on making consistent efforts towards your goals.

Setting a goal of 1% improvement daily is the best thing we can do for ourselves. It's all about understanding that consistent small improvements lead to big results in the long run. Instead of feeling overwhelmed and trying to achieve everything at once, focus on laying one brick at a time to build a strong foundation of good habits. For instance, if you take a few minutes each day to declutter and get rid of unnecessary items, your home will gradually become clutter-free. Instead of trying to clean the whole house at once, focus on one area at a time and organize it in a way that it stays tidy. By doing this consistently, you'll end up with a clean and organized home. We'll discuss goal-setting in more detail in the upcoming chapter.

Achieving your goal can be done in just two steps.

First, it's important to clearly define what you want to accomplish.

Second, create a system that works for you and take small actions each day towards your goal. With dedication and consistency, you'll be surprised at what you can achieve!

By setting a minimal target for yourself, you can overcome resistance and achieve your goals more easily. For example, if you want to cut down on your sugar intake, try taking one less sip of your coffee each day. If you need to read a boring but important book, start with a goal of reading just two pages each day. Starting small will help you stay motivated and make it easier to reach your ultimate goal. As you become more comfortable with the process, you can gradually increase your efforts until you reach your desired outcome.

Learning to ask yourself the right questions can make all the difference in achieving your goals. Instead of asking yourself a daunting question like "how can I read this entire book?", which can easily lead to procrastination and excuses, try shrinking the question down to something more manageable. For example, ask yourself "what's the very next thing I can do?" or "what's just one thing I can do to get started?". This small step approach helps you to start and gain momentum towards your goal. Starting is often the most difficult phase of completing a task, and setting a minimal target can help you overcome this hurdle and build the habit of daily progress towards your goal. Remember, small consistent steps lead to big improvements over time.

To improve in that area and take one small action towards it. Remember, it's not about taking giant leaps or achieving big goals overnight, but it's about making consistent small improvements every day. If you improve by just 1% each day you will be 100 % better in 100 days. Find out where we need to improve in our lives. It could be in terms of knowledge, spirituality, health, or any other aspect. Before you know it, you will have made significant progress and achieved your desired outcome. Celebrate your progress, no matter how small, and keep moving forward towards your goal.

Contrary to what most motivational speakers proclaim, taking big bold steps is not the only way to achieve great things. While it may seem exciting at the moment, the excitement quickly wears off when we realize how much work is involved. This can lead to fear, stress, and anxiety, which in turn can result in procrastination and distractions like TV and Facebook. Taking small actions consistently is a better approach and helps to lay the foundation for new positive habits. By following the philosophy of this Hadith, your resistance to change weakens and you will improve every day. With slow but steady progress, you will eventually reach your desired goal as long as you keep your momentum going.

Ask yourself, "What's the tiniest step I can take to move towards my goal?"

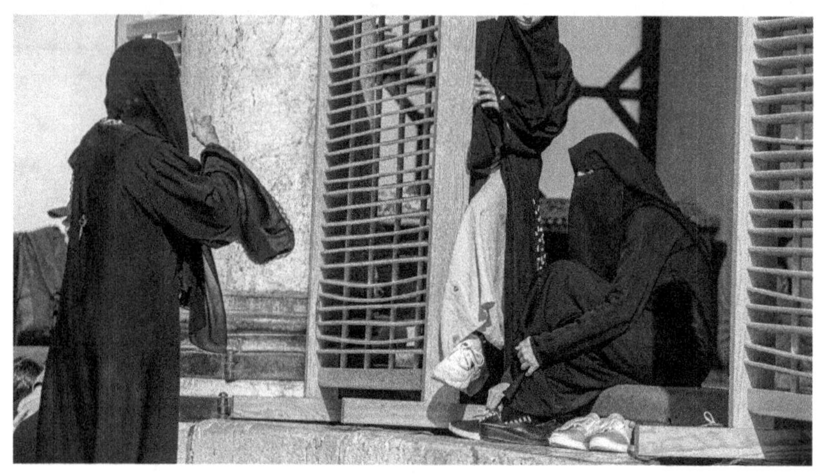

5 MINUTES CHALLENGE TO GET THINGS DONE

"WORK EXPANDS SO AS TO FILL THE TIME AVAILABLE
FOR ITS COMPLETION". PARKINSON'S LAW

Starting a task can be a real challenge, and we all know how tough it is to motivate ourselves to do something, whether it's cleaning, writing, or working on a project. Without a deadline, it's easy to procrastinate and put things off until the last minute. I bet you've been in that situation where you want to rearrange that one corner in your living room, but keep putting it off until you have guests coming over. Or when you have a project with a three-month deadline, but only start working on it a week before it's due. Don't worry sister, I've got a solution for you! It's called the 5-

Minute Challenge, and it's a great way to get started and get the ball rolling. Take a deep breath, and let's get started!

Let's learn the rules of the game:

-Choose a task you want to complete
-Set a timer for 5 minutes
-Try to do as much as you can in five minutes.

The way it works is a mystery, you will know when you give it a shot. Keep me posted on what you discover!

[Take the first step]

WHY NOT INVOLVE YOUR KIDS IN THE 5-MINUTE
CHALLENGE GAME? IT CAN BE A FUN WAY TO GET THINGS
DONE WHILE SPENDING QUALITY TIME WITH THEM.
ASSIGN DIFFERENT TASKS TO EACH CHILD, SET THE
TIMER, AND GET READY, SET, GO!

Then there is 20 minutes to increase your focus. Coming up Pomodoro technique

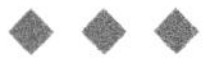

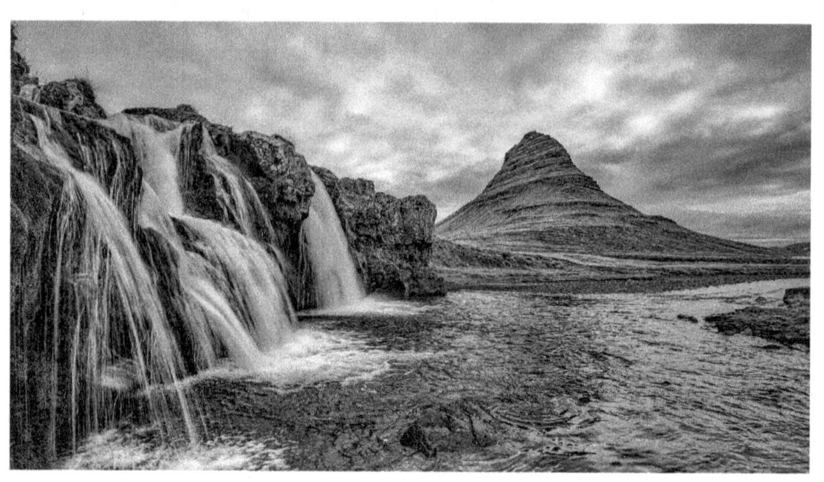

SMALL HABITS, BIG **STREAMS** OF REWARDS

One of the easiest ways to earn rewards is by cultivating small habits that can automate good deeds. For instance, you can try saying "Subhan Allah" and "Alhamdulillah" for every mentionable thing. This way, you can earn rewards throughout the day and soothe your heart by constantly remembering Allah. Additionally, it can help you avoid negative emotions such as guilt, fear, and anxiety. When you are preoccupied with the remembrance of Almighty, you will also refrain from indulging in vain and unnecessary talk that can often lead to negative emotions.

Prophet muhammad peace be upon him said "Whoever believes in Allah and the Last Day, let him speak goodness or remain silent." Sahih Muslim 47

"May Allah purify our tongue from unnecessary talk"

Have you ever wondered why we can spend hours scrolling through social media but struggle to spend just 10 minutes reading the Quran? There are two main reasons for this.

Firstly, we associate social media and TV with **happiness** and joy, but in the long run, we may realize that we have wasted a lot of time on something that doesn't bring us any real benefit.

Secondly, it's much easier to access social media and our smartphones than it is to access the Quran. Social media icons flash at us every time we unlock our phone, whereas the Quran icon may be hidden amongst other apps.

But if you ever decide to make a change, you'll find it's easier and more rewarding than you think.

Do you know what a habit is?

Habits are basically memories of steps that we took to solve a problem in the past. We use these memories to automatically apply the same solution when faced with a similar problem in the future. You don't even have to think about it; your mind does it automatically, like being on autopilot. For example, when you first learned to drive a car, you had to figure out where the gas pedal was and put in effort to remember it. But after a few days, it became automatic and you no longer had to consciously think about it.

Let's create new streams of rewards!
Growing small good habits is easier than you think. Just follow these three simple steps: (with a little bit of willpower and accountability, you can turn these small steps into valuable rewards)

-Choose the action you want to turn into a habit.
-Stack it with an action you already do as a habit.
-Repeat it consciously as much as you can.

Remember, any repetitive action can become a habit, so pay attention to your behavior. If you find yourself repeating the same action at the same time or situation, it could be the start of a new habit.

It's important to have patience when trying to develop a new habit. You won't see noticeable improvements or changes until you've passed the initial phase, so be sure to start with a small action and do it consistently. Don't fall into the trap of high enthusiasm in the beginning, only to have it taper off shortly after. Take it easy and make it effortless, as that approach is more likely to work. And don't try to perfect your habit right away; just focus on getting it to stick.

Start small and make it simple. Let's say you understand the benefits of daily journaling and want to implement it. If you expect yourself to write too much, it quickly feels like a chore. The key is to stay below the point where it feels like a simple job. In the beginning, keep a journal of **happiness**. Keep a small notepad and pen at your bedside and make a few notes about the good things which happened that day or the things you liked. Remember to thank Allah for every thing that you write down, it will help you cultivate a sense of gratitude and positivity in your life.

-If you want to start drinking water on an empty stomach in the morning, keep a glass of water at your bedside or somewhere visible before you start your morning routine.

-If you want to dedicate more time to reading the Quran, keep a copy of the Quran at your bedside and in the living room, where you spend most of your time. Keep the Quran icon on your smartphone's home screen and move the rest of the apps to the app screen. Additionally, frequently change the location of your most-used social media app icon and keeping the Quran icon in a prominent place, making it easier to access the Quran and delaying the temptation to access social media.

-For healthier eating habits, try serving yourself a small portion of veggies first, even if it's only a spoonful.

-If you want to wake up an hour earlier, set an alarm and when it goes off, get up and sleep on the couch for an hour. Do this for a few days, and after a while, start watching your favorite show or series while lying down on the couch. Your body will eventually adapt to this new routine, and it will be easier to wake up an hour earlier. Once you've established this habit, start scheduling activities to do during that extra hour.

Remember that it's okay to miss a day when trying to establish a new habit, but never miss two days in a row, as it can lead to losing progress. The duration of the habit-forming process depends on repetition and consistency.

Have you heard of habit stacking? It's a simple but effective way to build new habits by attaching them to existing ones. For instance, if you want to learn 3 Ayats per day from the Quran, you can stack it with your daily Salah routine. Just after finishing Salah, make a commitment to read 3 Ayats.

Here are some suggestions to get you started with habit stacking:
-Say Bismillah before starting dinner
-Meditate for 3 minutes while making coffee
-Perform ablution (Wudu) before getting into bed
-Listen to the Quran for 3 minutes before falling asleep
-Call a friend or relative to enquire about their health after finishing Zuhar Salah on Fridays

Remember, the key is to make your new habit small and easy to do. By stacking it with an existing habit, you can create a trigger that will help you remember to do it. Give it a try and see how it works for you!

Exchange all my bad habits with a good one

Have you ever thought about how amazing it would be if you could replace all your bad habits with good ones? We all have habits like mindless spending, excessive use of social media, or unhealthy eating habits that we know are not good for us. But it's hard to break free from them and develop better ones. Don't worry, we've got some simple tricks that can help you turn your bad habits into good ones.

(Please note that we are not referring to any kind of

drug or alcohol addiction here.)

Delay temptation

Delaying temptation can be an effective strategy to break bad habits and develop new ones. For instance, if you're trying to reduce your social media usage, you can place the Quran icon next to the call icon on your home screen. Whenever you feel the urge to check social media, read three Ayets from the Quran first. It won't take much time, and the results might surprise you.

You can also delay temptation by asking yourself two simple questions:
-What benefit will I get from it?
-How will it affect me in the long run?
By doing so, you can make a more informed decision and avoid giving in to impulsive urges. Give it a try and see how it works for you. By doing this, you can make your action more intentional rather than automatic.

If you often find yourself constantly checking your phone and want to break this habit, here's a simple trick that might help. Try disabling the fingerprint access and set a difficult P@s$w0rd to type. This way, when you feel the urge to check your phone unnecessarily, the trouble of typing in a complicated password might put you off or while unlocking the phone, you will have time to make a conscious choice instead of an automated, unconscious action. Don't worry if you struggle to stop yourself from bad habits at first. Just keep trying sincerely and pray to Allah. Your willpower will surely win over your bad habits someday.

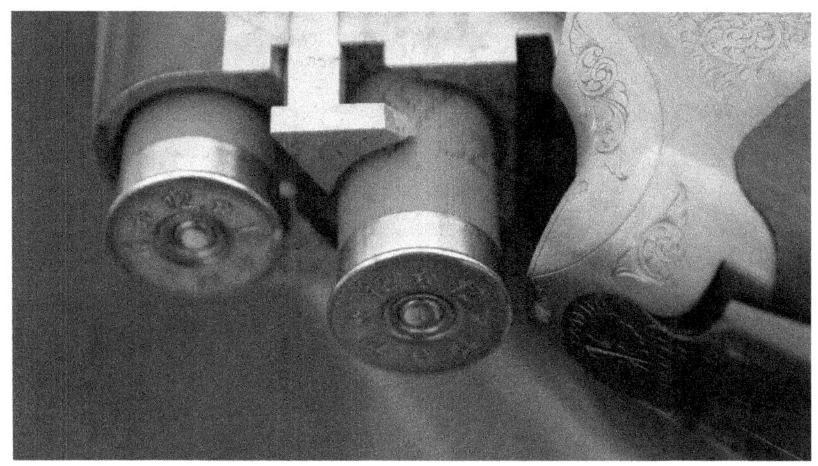

Eliminating **Triggers** To Help Break Bad Habits

If you enter a fast food restaurant for lunch, you are more likely to choose an unhealthy option compared to carrying a healthy lunch box with you.

Triggers! We all have them, and they can lead us astray from our good habits. For example, having your phone next to you while studying can make it tempting to check your social media (*try moving it to another room for better focus!*). Or having the TV remote next to you on the couch can make it too easy to channel surf (*moving it away from your living area can help you cut down on TV time*).

And we all know how tempting those checkout counter cookies can be when we're waiting in line at the grocery store! One way to resist the temptation is to make a list before you go shopping and stick to it. And if you remember something you forgot to put on the list, ask yourself if you can do without it for a week.

It's also important to be mindful of the company we keep.

For example, being around smokers can make it harder to quit, and having an obese friend can make it more difficult to maintain a healthy weight.

So, let's get rid of those small triggers that can spark unwanted behaviors. By recognizing and avoiding them, we can take control of our habits and make positive changes in our lives!

Motivate yourself by taking up a challenge.

If you have started a new diet plan, or are trying to finish reading a book or learn a new language, try announcing it on your social media, or tell your friends, spouse or family member. *For me, telling my kids does the job as kids are a constant reminder of my shortcomings.* This will put your reputation at stake and make it difficult for you to back down. You will put in extra effort to save face and accomplish your goals.

[Take the first step]

WAKE UP ONE HOUR EARLIER THAN USUAL AND SLEEP ON THE COUCH .

To sum up

Developing habits is a part of our daily lives, and we create and break them continually. To prevent ourselves from forming bad habits, it's crucial to recognize and halt them at the initial stage. If you notice yourself repeatedly watching the same thing at a specific time or repeatedly tapping on the same icon while unlocking your phone, it could be a sign that you are developing a new habit. Keep a check on your behavior and try to stop it at the beginning stage. If you find yourself engaging in repetitive behavior, identify what triggers the behavior and eliminate it.

*May **Allah** help me develop positive habit and protect us from harmful habits and addictions.*

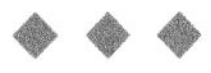

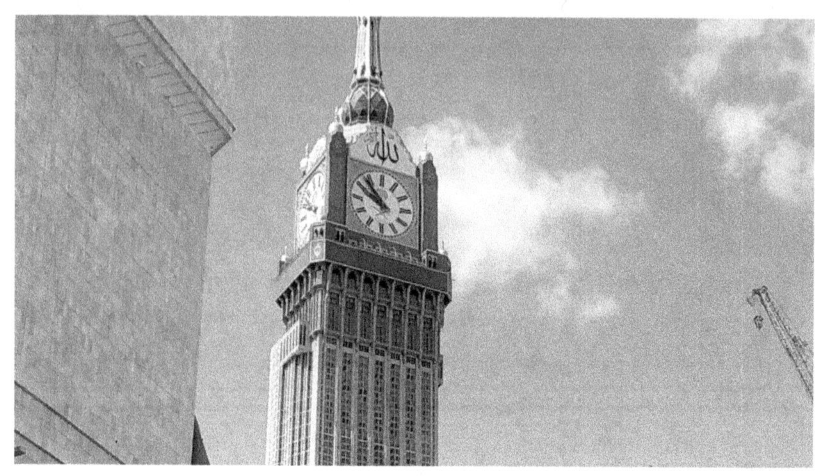

MANAGING YOURSELF: THE KEY TO EFFECTIVE **TIME** MANAGEMENT

"TAKE ADVANTAGE OF FIVE MATTERS BEFORE FIVE OTHER MATTERS: YOUR YOUTH BEFORE YOU BECOME OLD; YOUR HEALTH, BEFORE YOU FALL SICK; YOUR WEALTH, BEFORE YOU BECOME POOR; YOUR FREE TIME BEFORE YOU BECOME PREOCCUPIED, AND YOUR LIFE, BEFORE YOUR DEATH." **[HADITH : MUSNAD IMAM AHMAD]**

Have you ever had a day where you feel like you've been busy all day but haven't accomplished anything? To avoid this, try planning your day ahead and prioritize important tasks over trivial ones that waste time. When we don't organize our day, things can easily get out of control and cause stress and frustration. But don't worry, by simply creating a plan and prioritizing important tasks, you can avoid feeling overwhelmed and achieve more. By the end of the day, you'll feel a sense of accomplishment and motivation, knowing you've made progress towards your goals.

We can't manage time, we can manage ourselves.

Managing time may seem like a daunting task, but the truth is, we can manage ourselves to make the most out of the time we have. Start by making a habit of planning your day ahead of time before going to bed. This way, you can prioritize your tasks and ensure that you are focusing on what's important. Keep track of your progress by journaling your daily activities. The feeling of satisfaction and **happiness** you get from crossing off completed tasks is unmatched. Small accomplishments at the end of a tiring and busy day can make a world of difference. *This will help you in growing habit of success.*

[In the upcoming chapter, we will be discussing the 80/20 rule, which will help you learn how to set priorities effectively.]

Plan Your Way to Success

Before going to bed list the three most important things you should do the next day. Keeping a daily journal is absolutely vital for your self- improvement, you can check your progress and change course if needed. *Remember "If you can't measure you can't improve".* At the end of the day strike out whatever you have achieved and take an account of your day by asking these two simple questions.

-Where did I spend most of my time?
-What did I achieve in the day?

[Take the first step]

> *As you prepare to go to bed tonight, take a moment to reflect on your progress. Ask yourself these important questions: "What steps have I taken to protect myself from the hellfire?", "What have I learned today?", "How have I taken care of my body and mind?", and "How have I strengthened my spiritual well-being?"*

Be conscious of how you spend your 24 hours and prioritize your responsibilities. Take note of activities that waste your time and make an effort to minimize or eliminate them. Keep a journal or log of your day to hold yourself accountable and identify areas for improvement. Look for creative ways to optimize your time, such as using public transportation to catch up on reading or listening to audiobooks during your commute. Consider outsourcing small tasks to free up more time for important activities. Remember, every minute counts towards a more productive and fulfilling day.

> *[In the upcoming chapter, I'll provide you with assistance in calculating the worth of your time per hour. This way, you'll be able to determine how much you can afford to pay to outsource certain tasks]*

Make the most of your waiting time at the clinic by

carrying good reading material with you. Resist the urge to use your smartphone as it can easily distract you from your original purpose.

Your time could easily slip away while scrolling through social media, getting caught up in your cousin's engagement, your friend's vacation, or your aunt's complicated Italian dish recipe, leaving you with an hour of wasted time. And eventually, you'll leave the clinic with a prescription, feelings of envy, and a drained phone battery.

The airport waiting lounge or hospital waiting area can be great places to connect with others. Consider keeping Islamic books with you to read in public, which could spark someone's interest and potentially lead to a conversation about Allah. You won't believe the satisfaction and contentment one can feel when sharing information about Islam with non-Muslims. If you have ever experienced it, you know the feeling is much better than any meditation session.

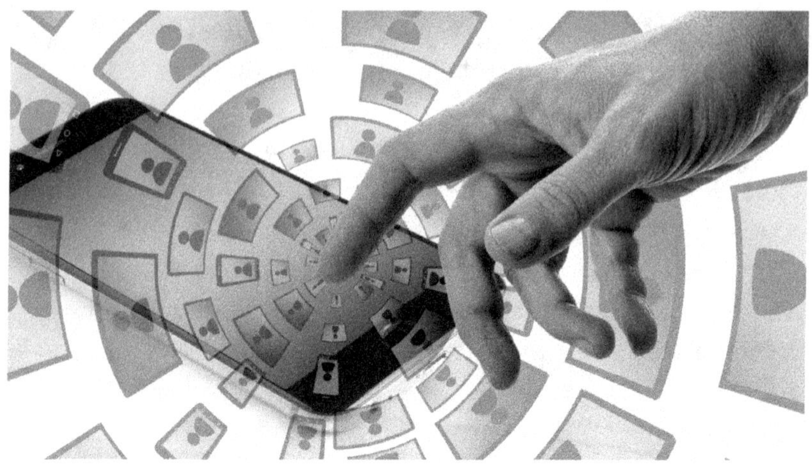

Never Too Busy To Prevent Future Interruptions And Distractions.

Eliminate anything that takes away your focus. For instance, suppose you are working on a project and receive a notification on your smartphone. You can't resist the temptation, so you check the message. One thing leads to another, and you end up spending 10-15 minutes checking and responding to irrelevant and non-urgent messages. You have already wasted your valuable time and focus on unimportant things. Spend 5 more minutes silencing the notification from that app, group, or person that took your precious attention away. Whenever you receive unwanted news, email, or video recommendations, block them before jumping into another interpretation. Investing a minute to block future interruptions and distractions can yield valuable returns.

[Take the first step]

Reflect and evaluate how you utilized your previous hour: Did you invest it wisely or squander it away?

◆ ◆ ◆

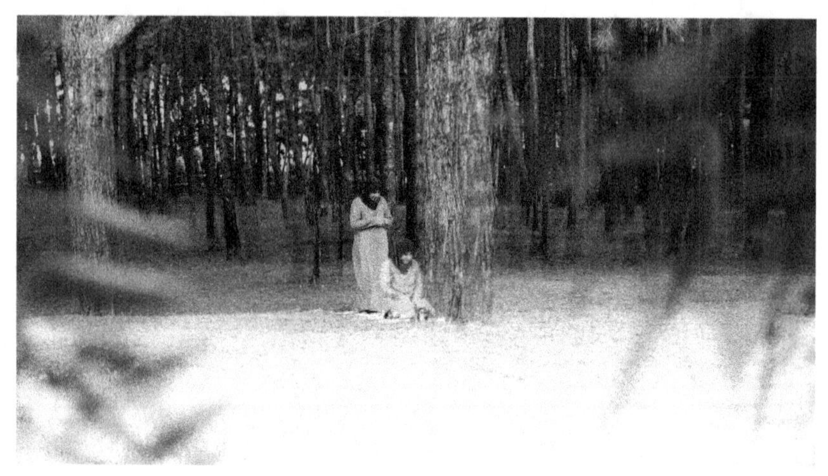

WHAT **REALLY** MATTERS TO YOU?

Prophet Muhammad (peace be upon him) said: "The feet of a servant will not move on the Day of Judgment until he is asked about his life and how he used it, his knowledge and what he did with it, his wealth and how he earned it and where he spent it, and his body and how he used it." (Tirmidhi)

It's easy to get caught up in the busyness of life and lose sight of what's important. Perceived **priorities** may differ from your actual priorities. By keeping track of where you spend most of your time and money, you can gain a better understanding of what your true priorities are. Don't worry if you discover that you're spending your life on the wrong and meaningless things. it's never too late to reset your priorities! Start by taking a look at where you're spending your time and money. Are they aligned with your values? If not, Here's a simple two-step plan to get you back on track:

1) Write down what your priorities should be.

2) Focus your time and money on those things.

"where your treasure is, there will your heart be also"

Have you ever heard of the **80/20 rule?** It's also known as the "rule of vital few." The idea is that roughly 20% of your efforts will produce 80% of your results. This doesn't mean it's a strict 20/80 split, but rather a general principle.

For example,
20% of the population controls 80% of the wealth,
20% of your wardrobe is worn 80% of the time, and
20% of your furniture at home is used 80% of the time.

This law can be observed in many areas of life. People who appear to be busy all day but accomplish very little Often, they are working on tasks that are low or no value and neglecting the truly important ones. So it's important to focus on the 20% of tasks that will produce 80% of the results, and not get bogged down in unimportant activities.

Let's talk about how we can implement the 80/20 rule in our daily lives.
It's a really useful principle that can be applied to goal-setting and productivity. Before starting your day, take a moment to ask yourself: What tasks are in the top 20%

of my activities? By doing this, you'll develop the habit of prioritizing the important things in your life.

Did you know that 85% of successful people have one big goal that they work on all the time?

So, write down ten tasks and then ask yourself: if I could only finish one of them, which one would have the greatest positive impact on my goal? Don't fall into the trap of clearing up small unimportant things first.

At the end of the day, use the chart below to check where you've been spending your time. Most of the daily activities can be classified into four quadrants to help you set your priorities. Tick the activities you've performed throughout the day

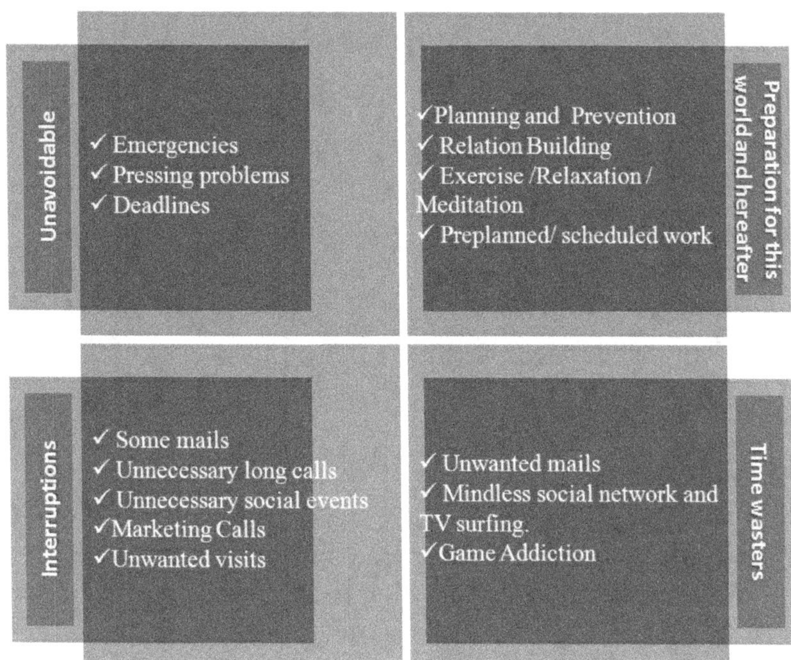

Inspired by 4 quadrants of time management by Stephen R. Covey's

[Take the first step]

> *list 10 tasks that you think are important to accomplish it. Then, cross out 8 of them and focus only on the two that you think will have the biggest impact. By accomplishing these two tasks, you'll be much closer to achieving your goal.* **Remember, taking small steps every day can lead to big results in the long run.**

Teach this to kids. You can help your kids by teaching them this rule early on. It can have a big impact on their life. For example when they're preparing for exams, encourage them to tackle the questions that carry the most marks first and give them their full attention before moving on to the questions with fewer marks. This will help them learn to prioritize their tasks and get the best results possible.

In conclusion, setting priorities is crucial for achieving success and living a fulfilling life. The 80/20 rule or the Pareto Principle can be a useful tool in identifying the most important tasks and focusing our time and energy on them. By regularly assessing our priorities and making conscious choices about how we spend our time and resources, we can work towards our goals and make the most of our lives. Whether we are young or old, prioritizing our activities is crucial not only for our productivity and success but also for our mental and spiritual well-being. Start your day by identifying the most important task you need to accomplish. At the end of the day, take some time to reflect on how you spent your time. Rather than wasting time on trivial activities that contribute little or nothing, focus on the 20% of activities that will have the greatest impact on your progress.

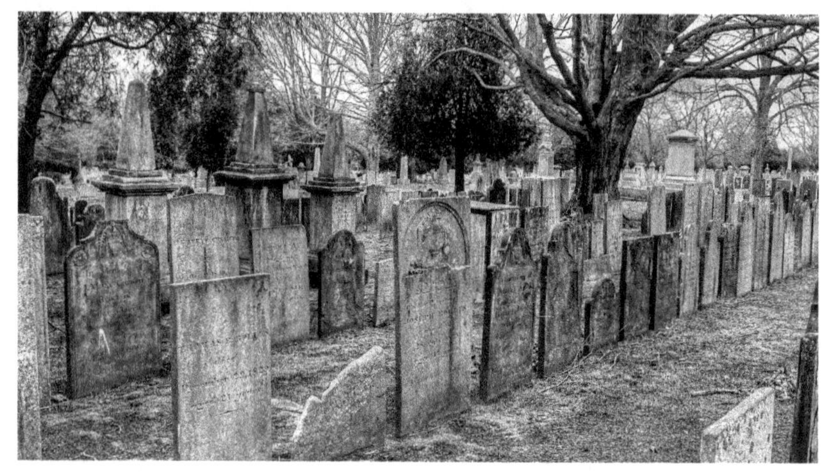

HOW KNOWING YOUR **WORTH** CAN CHANGE YOUR LIFE?

Have you ever wondered how much your time is truly worth? You can calculate the value of your hour by dividing your total earnings by the total number of hours you work. But let me give you a fun way to think about it. If you could talk to a departed loved one and ask them how much they would pay for just one more hour of life, even if they owned all the world's wealth, their answer would give you an idea of the true value of your time.

[The typical number of pages in a standard Arabic printed Quran is around 604, to complete reading the entire Quran in 30 days, you can read just 4 pages before or after each obligatory salah.]

It is important to consider how we invest our time in order to improve our lives in both this world and the next. Rather than comparing ourselves to unrealistic social media images, we should focus on competing in good deeds. There are many apps and groups that can help us learn and grow, and even small amounts of time can be used productively. By organizing our time and cutting out time-wasting activities, we can gain valuable extra hours in our day. Remember, even saving one minute a day can add up to an extra hour in just 60 days, which is more valuable than any amount of gold. ***So take a deep breath, prioritize your time, and start investing in yourself ,in future and in your Akhirah (the Hereafter).***

[Did you know that it's possible to learn a new language on an intermediate level with just a few minutes of practice per day? It's true! All you need is to learn around 400 commonly used words, and you'll be able to communicate effectively in that language. If you break it down, that's less than 5 words per day over a period of 90 days. By dedicating just 20-30 minutes of practice each day, you can achieve this goal in as little as 3 months.]

CONSERVE YOUR BRAIN **ENERGY**

Have you ever felt tired and drained of energy even though you haven't done anything physically demanding? It could be because you're making too many small decisions throughout the day. Simple things like choosing what to wear or what to eat for breakfast can take up valuable mental energy that you could be using to focus on more important tasks. That's why it's important to streamline your life and eliminate as many unnecessary decisions as possible. By doing so, you can preserve your energy for the things that truly matter and avoid wasting it on trivial matters.

Why some famous people wear the same clothes every day?

You may have heard of people like Mark Zuckerberg of Facebook or ex-president Barack Obama doing this. The reason for this is actually quite interesting - it's to make fewer decisions! As the day goes on, the quality of our decision-making tends to deteriorate, so by wearing the same thing every day, we free up mental space for more important decisions. Plus, it saves time and **energy** that would otherwise go into picking out outfits and taking care of a larger wardrobe. It's not necessarily about wearing the exact same shirt or pair of underwear every single day, but rather having multiples of the same outfit. Pretty cool, right?

Don't waste your first decision of the day

Let's focus our brain power on what really matters and take steps to make our lives easier and less stressful. That way, we can make the most of each day and feel good about the positive impact we're making on the world around us. We're lucky to have the opportunity to make a positive impact on those around us every day, and it's our responsibility to prioritize our efforts towards building the best versions of ourselves and our loved ones.

When it comes to decision-making, it's easy to get overwhelmed and exhaust ourselves. That's why it's helpful to plan ahead and organize our lives as much as possible. By arranging things like our wardrobe in advance, we can save ourselves from the stress of making small decisions like what to wear or what to cook for dinner. This means you have less stress in the morning.

Our brain is actually an incredible analytical and creative machine, rather than just a **memory storage device.** Unfortunately, many of us tend to overload our brains by trying to remember too many things at once. But the good news is that we don't have to rely solely on our brains to keep track of everything. Thanks to technology, we can use our mobile devices as a handy tool for remembering important tasks and events. Use mobile calendar to plan ahead, set reminders, and make notes. This can help take the burden off our brains and allow us to focus on *our analytical and creative skills* instead. Give brains a break by using technology and utilizing the **extended memory**. By doing so, we can free up our minds to think more deeply and creatively, which can lead to some amazing ideas and solutions.

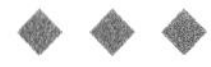

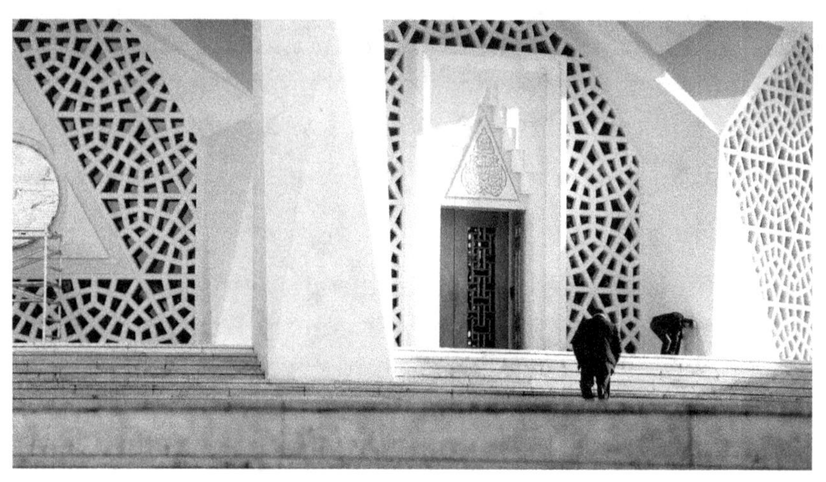

SIMPLICITY AND **HAPPINESS**: HOW LESS CAN TRULY BE MORE

Have you noticed how the definition of "the good life" seems to revolve around having the latest gadgets, trendy clothes, expensive decor, and being popular on social media? It's almost like we're falling into a trap of bank debt just to keep up appearances. But let's pause for a moment and take a *deeeep breath*. Even with all of these material possessions, we can't truly be happy. In fact, we're cluttering our lives with excess stuff that doesn't bring us genuine joy. It's like we know that consumerism isn't the answer to our **happiness**, but we feel helpless because society seems to praise over-consumption. The mindless shopping we engage in leaves us with cluttered lives that only add burden to our minds.

It's ironic how we've started to love stuff and use people, when it should be the other way around. Let's strive to find **happiness** in simpler things and focus on what truly matters in life.

> DO NOT BE A WASTEFUL SPENDER. SQUANDERERS ARE
> THE BROTHERS OF SATAN. SATAN WAS FAITHLESS TO HIS
> LORD. QURAN (17:27)

Have you ever thought about simplifying your life and getting rid of unnecessary stuff? It's time to throw out social norms and make room for more meaningful things in your life. Start by identifying what's truly essential and let go of the rest. I know you may have spent money on these things, but your freedom is much more valuable than any material possession. You'll be left with more authentic and worthwhile things and much more space to live. **Minimalism.**

It's a philosophy that reflects the teachings of the Quran, as quoted above. It's all about simplifying your journey and getting back to the basics of what's truly important in your life. Minimalism helps you take back control of your own life, time, money, and energy, by rejecting the idea that material possessions are the key to **happiness** and fulfillment.

You don't have to strip yourself of every single thing in your life to be a minimalist. The idea is to really think about what brings value to your life. Minimalism is a reminder that you are not defined by what you have. Life can be so freeing when you focus on what really matters.

Remember the 80/20 rule?

Clear space, clear mind. Use minimalism as a tool to change your life. Ask yourself if something is absolutely necessary or if it adds value to your life. Cut back on the apps you have on your phone to only what you need, and reduce the time you spend mindlessly scrolling through social media or watching TV.

Start by selling, donating, or recycling things that don't add value to your life. You don't have to declutter everything overnight, as that's not always possible. It's an ongoing and lifelong process that requires taking it one step at a time. You can improve bit by bit, day by day, and eventually, you'll see significant progress. It may take months or years to become a minimalist, but taking it slow will help you avoid accidentally getting rid of something you need.

Of course, minimalism doesn't apply to documentation. Be careful with important papers, instead of keeping hard copies, scan and email them to yourself, so that you can access them while traveling. Take digital photos of sentimental items as a way to remember them before throwing away old stuff. Remember that decluttering is an ongoing process, so keep up the good work, and eventually, you'll see the benefits of a simpler and more intentional lifestyle.

Experiences are worth more than things

We often fall prey to impulsive purchases and the temptation of buying new stuff. But let's ask ourselves: what brings more joy and satisfaction in life, material possessions or experiences? Take a moment to reflect on your childhood memories: are they about the things you had or the experiences you shared?

Before making a purchase, let's practice restraint and hold off for at least a month. We might find that we don't actually need it, or that life goes on just fine without it. Be mindful of the language used in advertisements, such as "Buy Now," "Offer Ends Today," and "Early-Bird Discount." These phrases are designed to create a sense of urgency and push us towards impulsive spending.

The next time we feel the urge to buy something, let's pause and ask ourselves a few questions:

Do I really need this?

Is it worth the money I've earned through hard work?

Could I use this money in better ways?

Becoming more mindful of your spending habits is a great way to make a positive impact on the environment and your budget. One way to do this is to prioritize quality over quantity. When you choose to invest in higher-quality pieces, you can expect them to last longer, reducing the need for frequent replacements. This not only saves you money in the long run, but it also helps reduce waste in your home and in the world.When you are in the market for a new item, take the time to research and compare products to find the best quality option within your budget. Look for items made from durable and sustainable materials, and consider purchasing from companies with a commitment to ethical and eco-friendly production methods. Remember that buying higher quality does not mean you have to spend a fortune. It's about choosing items that are well-made, functional, and align with your values. By prioritizing quality over quantity, you can create a more intentional and sustainable lifestyle.

How to start being minimalist?

To start being minimalist, it's important to take small steps and not expect to become minimalist overnight. One approach is to take a box and fill it with broken or useless items around your home every day for a week or so. Once you can't find any more of those items, start filling the box with things you think you can manage without. After a month, revisit the box and consider what can still be of value to you and dispose of the rest through selling, donating or throwing them away.

When it comes to children's items, be patient and respectful of their emotional attachment to their belongings. Similarly, be mindful of older people who may not be open to the idea of minimalism. Remember, being a minimalist does not mean you have to live miserably or define a specific item limit. Instead, focus on getting rid of items that you can live without and strive to live a modest life *without making a show of your minimalism.*

Living a modest life can indeed be a blessing. By being mindful of our spending habits and avoiding the temptation to constantly buy new things, we can save a lot of money and reduce waste. For example, the average American family spends a significant amount of money on clothing each year, much of which goes unused and eventually gets thrown away. By downsizing and resisting the urge to constantly consume, we can not only save money, but also free up space in our homes and reduce our impact on the environment.

Instead of prioritizing material possessions, we can focus on experiences and helping others. By saving money and investing in experiences like travel, we can create lasting memories and enrich our lives in ways that material goods cannot. Additionally, we can use our resources to support those in need and make a positive impact on the world around us.

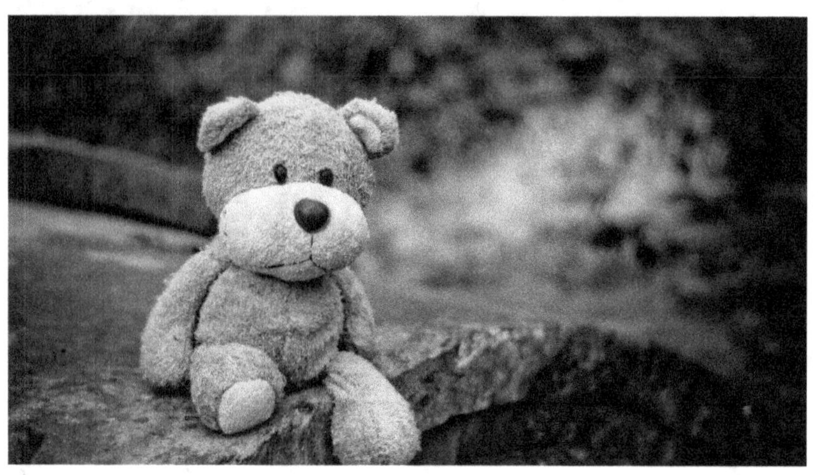

BALANCE BETWEEN AMBITION AND **GRATITUDE**

"If you give thanks, I will certainly grant you more; but if you are ungrateful for My favours, My chastisement is terrible" **Quran 14:7**

You know what's wrong with the way we set goals these days? We tend to think that achieving our goals is the key to **happiness** and success, but that's not always true. When we fall short, we end up feeling disappointed and discouraged. Instead of just focusing on the end result, let's try to enjoy the journey and celebrate every little progress we make towards our goal. Remember, even if things don't turn out exactly as planned, you're still making progress and that's something to be proud of. Goals can sometimes make us feel stuck, so let's not let them define our **happiness**. Achieving a goal might make us happy for a moment, but it won't necessarily solve all our problems.

Sometimes we get so caught up in achieving our goals that we forget to enjoy the journey along the way. Have you ever worked super hard towards a goal, only to feel disappointed when you didn't get the exact outcome you wanted? It can be tough! But here's the thing - the result of your actions is your fate, and it's important to accept it with gratitude (Alhamdulillah!).

Take studying for a big exam, for example. It's easy to get so focused on getting the highest score that we forget to enjoy the learning process. And sometimes, even if we do well, we might realize that the journey towards the goal wasn't really worth it. That's why it's important to set goals that align with our values and faith, and to always remember to be grateful for whatever outcome we receive.

Set goals, but remember to enjoy the process along the way. And if the outcome isn't exactly what you hoped for, embrace it with gratitude and keep moving forward. Trust me, with a little patience and practice, you'll find joy and **happiness** in each day, rather than just at the finish line.

"O you who have believed, avoid much [negative] assumption. Indeed, some assumption is sin." Quran 49:12

Don't Believe Everything You Think

Our brains are always working overtime, filling our heads with unwanted and irritating thoughts that make us anxious and negative about ourselves, situations, and other people. Most of these negative feelings are based on assumptions. Like, "What will people think of me?" "Will my kids ever make it big?" "Am I going to be a failure forever?" "I just know something bad is going to happen!" We worry about our future, even though we have no control over it, and we regret our past, which we can't change.

But here's the thing: Our thoughts have the power to influence our emotions and mental state in a big way. So, if we can learn to control our thoughts, we can manage our anger, depression, anxiety, guilt, and all the other negative feelings that bring us down. And one way to do that is through meditation. *By focusing on the signs of Allah and His blessings, we can guide our thoughts towards positivity and peace.*

Guilt of being happy

Have you ever had a moment during a busy day where you suddenly feel happy, but then you start questioning why you feel that way and try to find reasons why you shouldn't be happy? It's like a debate starts inside your head and you convince yourself that there must be something to worried about. You end up going back to your usual state of worry and guilt. But if this ever happens to you again, just remember that feeling happy and content is a blessing from Allah. So don't let those negative thoughts take away from that moment of joy.

S m i l e and say الْحَمْدُ لِلَّهِ, *(Alhamdulillah) and promise yourself that you will give a little bit of Sadaqa (charity)*

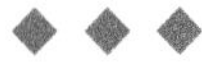

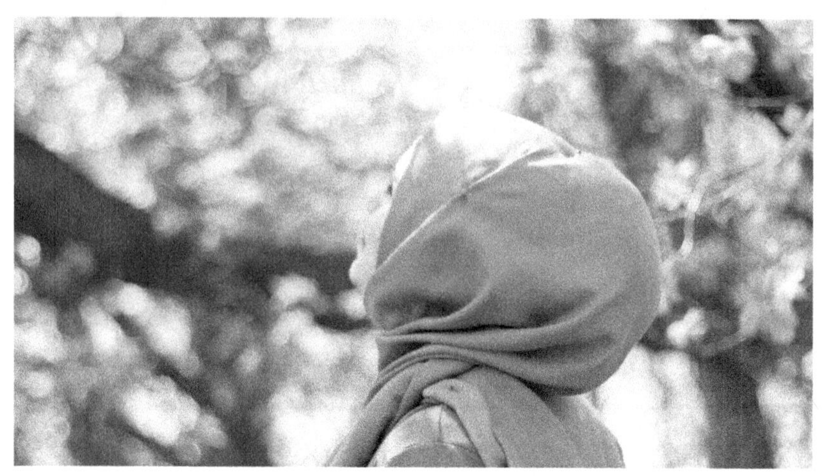

GRATITUDE

"All praise is due to Allah who has given us life after causing us to die and to Him is the return." (Bukhari)

It's a beautiful reminder of the gift of life we've been given, yet we often spend our days chasing material possessions and neglecting our health and spirituality. ***May Allah protect us from this path.*** We make lengthy wish lists, but forget to express gratitude for the blessings we already have. As humans, we're known for our ingratitude, even though the favors of Allah are countless and immeasurable. We all know this, but we often fail to appreciate it.

And [remember] when your Lord proclaimed, 'If you are grateful, I will surely increase you [in favor]; but if you deny, indeed, My punishment is severe.'

"Quran 14:7

Developing the habit of saying *Alhamdulillah* and expressing gratitude through our actions is crucial for finding true **happiness** in life. One way to show gratitude is by giving in charity, being kind and smiling towards others, and maintaining good character. Remember, gratitude is essential to **happiness,** and there is nothing more damaging to our *peace* and tranquility than being ungrateful towards Allah. So, always remember to smile and thank Allah for all the blessings He has bestowed upon you.

I will leave you with a small story; I forget where I have heard it.

> *Once, a man was on his way back home from work feeling exhausted and unfulfilled. Along the way, he saw a homeless man and thought to himself, "Thank God I am not homeless." The homeless man, in turn, saw a woman begging for food and said, "Thank God I am not hungry." Just then, an ambulance rushed past them, and the woman said, "Thank God I am not sick." When the sick person arrived at the hospital, they saw a dead body of a young man and said, "Thank God I am not dead." It is only the dead who cannot thank **Allah** for His blessings.*

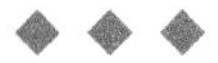

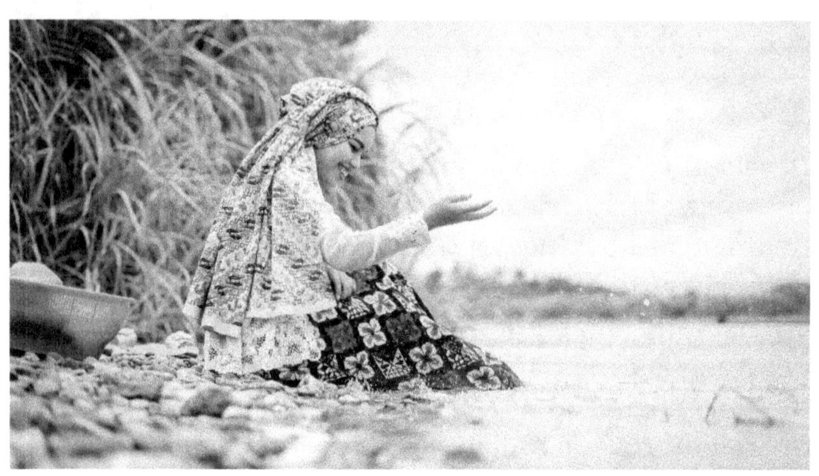

POSITIVE THINKING

"And when My servants ask you concerning Me, then (answer them), I am indeed near to them. I respond to the invocations of the supplicant when he calls on Me!" AL-Quran

Life is a precious gift from Allah, and we should not waste it in worries and negative thoughts. Instead, we should look at everything with a positive mindset and always keep our focus on the Hereafter. We must do our best in every action we take and leave the result to Allah, for He knows what is best for us. Even if the outcome is not what we expected, we should avoid doubts and have good expectations from Allah, the Most Merciful. We should always make sincere dua and ask Allah for the best outcome.

It is important to have good expectations from Allah as it shows our trust in Him. Amongst the etiquette of Dua is to expect the best from Allah. If a person only expects good from Allah, Allah will not destroy his hopes." So, let us always have faith in Allah and expect the best from Him.

"Ask Allah for everything, even the lace of a shoe .." (Hadith)

To make the best decision, it's important to take all available measures and seek guidance from knowledgeable individuals. Don't forget to pray Salat-al-Istikhara and ask Allah for guidance before taking any action. And once you have decided on your course of action, put your trust in Allah by saying "Twakkul Ala Allah".

The true loss is the loss in the Hereafter, so it's essential to always keep that in mind. Instead of having doubts, have good expectations from Allah and perform good deeds with the hope of receiving the best reward in both worlds. Remember, every hardship in this world will be rewarded in the Aakhirah.

"And whoever relies upon Allah - then He is sufficient for him." Quran 65:2

MAY ALLAH MAKE THINGS EASY FOR US.

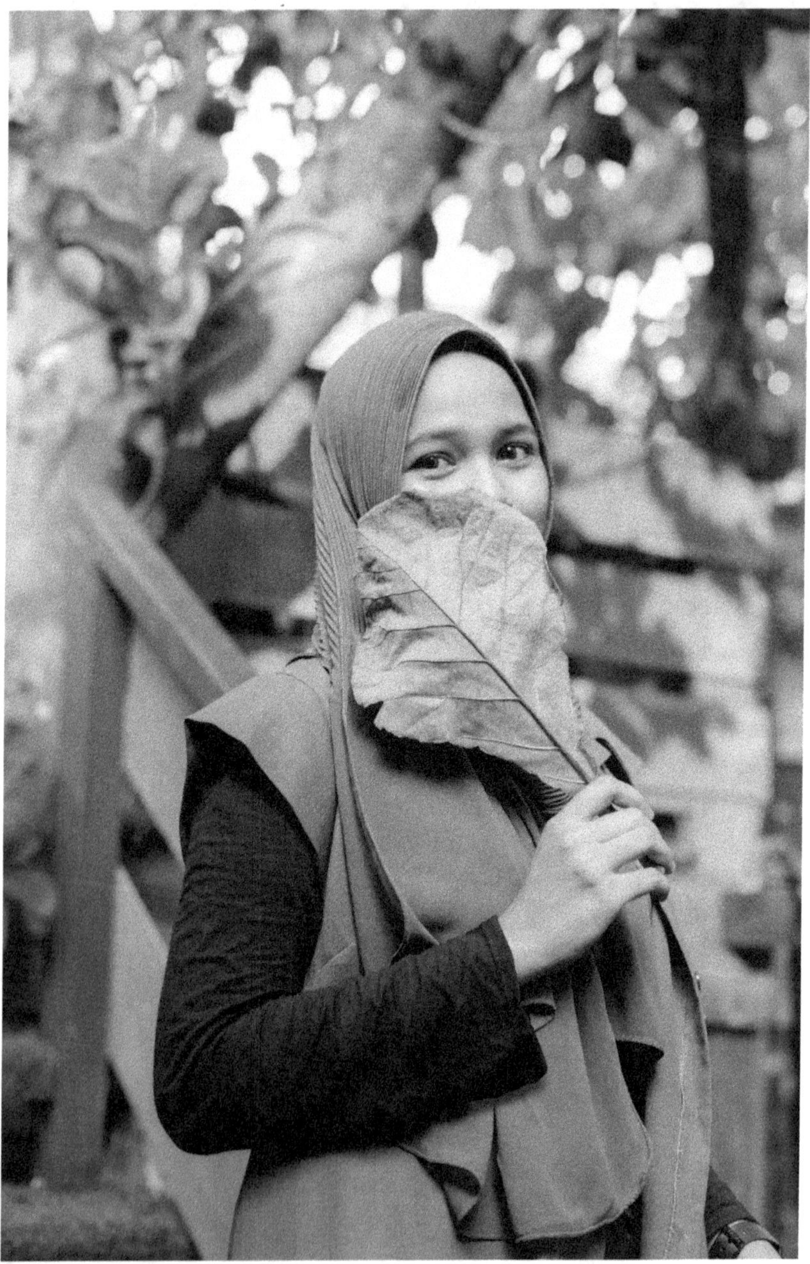

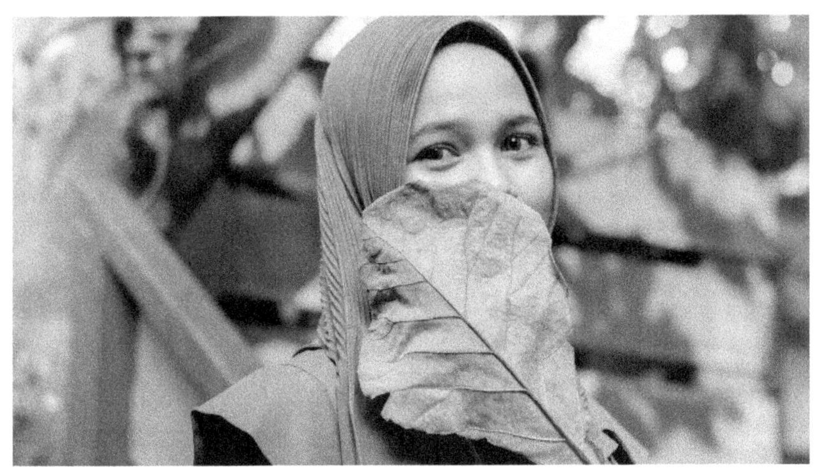

CAN MONEY TRULY BUY *HAPPINESS*?

The worth of money is not determined by the amount but rather by the unmet needs and desires of an individual. A hungry and homeless person may only yearn for food, while a middle-class individual may focus on paying their bills. Meanwhile, a wealthy individual may strive for even more luxuries such as new gadgets, expensive cars, lavish furniture or to accumulate more wealth.

There are individuals who may appear wealthy by purchasing extravagant gadgets and luxury items on credit card. They might look rich but It is different than being really rich.

Changing Your Perspective

The cost of the device you're using to read this book could actually provide basic supplies for someone in need for several months

Instead of always chasing after the latest smartphone or luxury car, take a moment to reflect on the value of your possessions. Think about how much the price of silver has appreciated since you bought your last expensive phone or car. Consider the benefits of investing in something that has the potential to earn you a return rather than just depreciating over time. I am not recommending investing in silver or any other specific commodity. Rather, I am presenting a different viewpoint for you to consider. Of course, earning halal income is a religious obligation, there is nothing wrong with investing or saving money wisely.

Investing in the Hereafter

"When a man dies, his deeds come to an end except for three things: Sadaqah Jariyah (ceaseless charity); a knowledge which is beneficial, or a virtuous descendant who prays for him (for the deceased)." (Muslim)

There is another better way; you can deposit your money in BOA (Bank of Akhrat) as a form of charity and earn rewards in the afterlife. Even better, invest in the Hereafter through **Sadaqah Jariyah**, which has a compounding effect and continues to benefit the donor even after their death.

Material possessions may provide temporary **happiness**, they cannot provide lasting contentment. Imagine having a bad headache - even if you're watching your favorite movie on the most expensive home theater, you will not be able to enjoy it. So, invest in things that will last forever and *buy peace with your hard-earned money.*

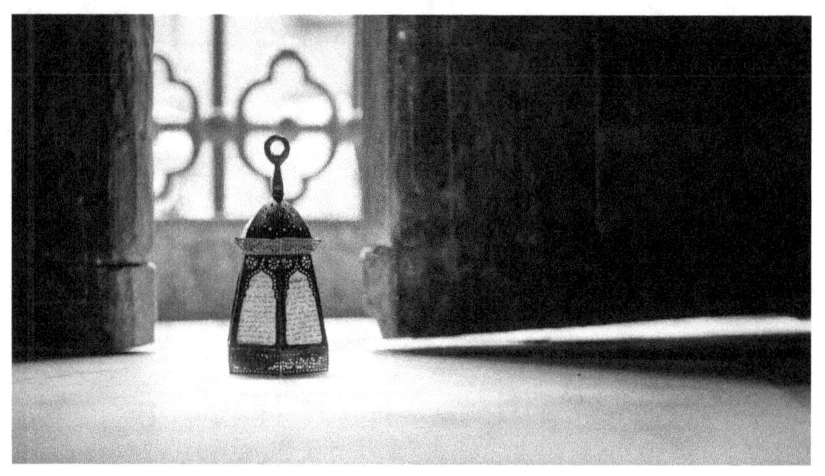

THE **FREEDOM** OF FORGIVENESS: RELEASE YOUR BURDENS

Imagine you're cruising down a busy road, minding your own business, when suddenly someone honks their horn, overtakes you, or starts hurling abuse at you for a mistake you didn't even realize you made. Your heart starts racing, your body tenses up, and your thoughts get derailed. You lose control of yourself.

Do you know what just happened? You're upset by someone you don't even know, and that person has no idea how much harm he has caused you. It's amazing how just a few words from a stranger can do so much damage. *So how can you shield yourself from the harmful impact of others' ignorance on your emotional well-being?*

Forgive and Flourish

"Those who give in times of both ease and hardship, those who control their rage and pardon other people , Allah loves the good-doers." (Qur'an, 3:134)

Anger can be more harmful to oneself than to others. It's no secret that it can damage our hearts. In fact, most of the time the other person may not even realize that we are angry or annoyed. The next time you feel angry, try taking a **deep breath** and offering a prayer for that person. The best time for making Dua is when you are hurt or angry, **(remember this during a trip to the dentist)**. Don't punish yourself for someone else's mistakes. There are plenty of foolish people in the world; don't become one of them. Keep your mind occupied with something of value, so that you can overlook the small things, and engage in the dhikr of Allah to attain inner **peace** When you hit the road, try to maintain a positive attitude and remind yourself that you're not there to find faults and punish others. Make it a habit to offer Dua to others instead of cursing them. When you pray for others, you're also praying for yourself, and it can help build your *character*. Finally, Make a beautiful deal with your Lord Almighty by forgiving the person and seeking forgiveness from Allah in return.

Do you believe that meditation or mindfulness can

*bring you the same level of **peace** as these practices?*

Don't curse

Whenever I get angry at someone and feel like cursing them, I ask Allah to give them a neighbor like themselves and me a neighbor like me. It makes me reflect on my own flaws and motivates me to improve my character, so that I can be someone who others enjoy living near. Do small things for your neighbor that only Allah knows, things like removing dry leaves from their car windshield, can purify your heart.

Remember that when you pray for your enemy, you are also praying for yourself. I pray for my most challenging neighbor's children, and I encourage my wife to do the same. I pray with sincerity, knowing that whatever I am asking for their kids, Allah will also grant to mine.

Here's a short story that highlights our selfish and foolish tendencies

There was a motel located on a busy highway and the owner was thriving due to the monopoly, resulting in a profitable business. One day, the owner's neighbor opened another motel on the opposite side of the road. To everyone's surprise, the new motel became an overnight success with no negative impact on the first one. However, the jealous wife of the first motel owner insisted that her husband do something about it because there was no traffic before they started and because of their motel people starting stopping there. After years of hard work, they were finally in a position to start earning a profit, and this new neighbor was reaping the benefits of their hard work.Feeling agitated, the motel owner went to a saint seeking advice. The saint told him that he could earn millions, provided that the new motel owner earned twice what he earned. The motel owner thought for a moment and asked the saint, "Will he get double of whatever I get?" The saint replied, "Yes, even calamity, pain, or loss." The motel owner paused for a moment, then said, "Blind me from one eye.

*The moral of the story is that we often prioritize the misery of others over our own **well-being.***

Reflect on your heart for a moment, is that not the case ? Do you make dua for others, including difficult neighbors or people you encounter on the road? Remember, even small acts of kindness can have a big impact on our own hearts and the wellbeing of our families.

The Prophet Muhammad (peace be upon him) said, "He who supplicates for his brother behind his back (in his absence), the Angel commissioned (for carrying supplication to his Lord) says: Amen, and it is for you also."

Instead of just focusing on breathing in and out on a yoga mat, try incorporating forgiveness and prayer into your daily routine for even greater inner **peace***.*

[Take the first step]
Close your eyes and say from the bottom of your heart that you have truly forgiven "that person". You will experience a sense of **peace** *and tranquility in your heart that is beyond compare to any benefits gained from meditation or mindfulness practices.*

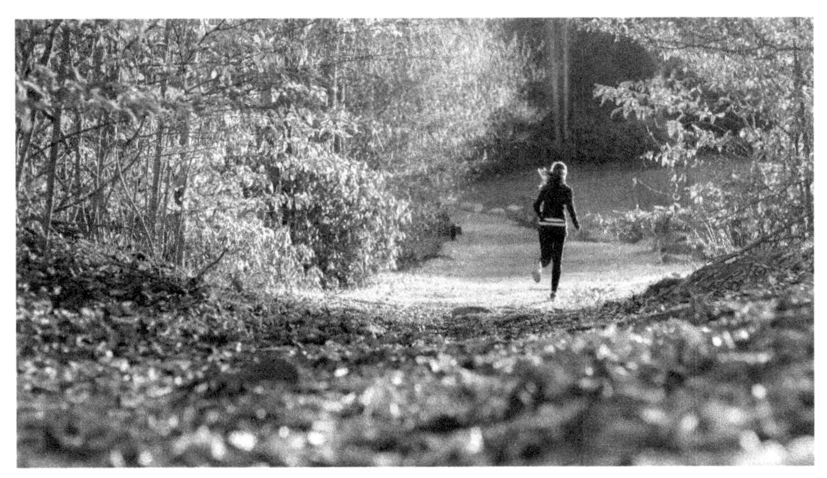

OVERCOMING **LAZINESS**: ISLAMIC PERSPECTIVES

Have you ever wondered how some people manage to accomplish so much in the same 24 hours we all have? It can be tough to motivate ourselves to work when we're feeling sluggish or unmotivated. Here are some valuable tips from an Islamic perspective to combat laziness:

-Resist the urge to yawn and cover your mouth when you do yawn.

-Avoid overeating and make sure to leave some space in your stomach for breathing, with one-third for food, one-third for water, and one-third empty.

-If you're surrounded by lazy people, distance yourself from them.

-Build up mental strength - sometimes we think we're tired, but we're not actually physically tired.

O Allah, I seek refuge in You from grief and sadness, from weakness and from laziness, from miserliness and from cowardice, from being overcome by debt and overpowered by men (i.e. others). (Al-Bukhari 7/158.)

Use **Kaizen** to fight laziness.

Take laziness as a challenge, give yourself small tasks. There is a Japanese technique to overcome laziness; it is called the **1-minute principle.** The idea is that you should practice doing something for a single minute every day at the same time, just for a minute no more.

Shouldn't be any trouble for absolutely anyone right? Even the laziest person can do it. We usually find an excuse not to do something when we are expected to carry out for thirty minutes or for an hour; however, we could not be able to find an excuse for not doing it for 60 seconds.

Why this method works ?

When starting a new activity, it can be challenging to find the energy to continue. It's common to feel demotivated at the beginning stage. This technique is so easy and doable that it doesn't feel like a burden to complete any task. Whether you're learning a new language or planning to do the dishes it won't seem unpleasant, instead after completing the exercise, you will experience a sense of satisfaction, contentment, and **happiness**,

Don't attempt to transform your life all at once. Instead, take one small step at a time, and you will make progress towards becoming a more energetic individual. This approach will assist you in overcoming low confidence, as you will feel a sense of accomplishment and gradually increase the amount of time you dedicate to your pursuits.

O Allah, make me among the happy, make me among the companions of the right hand, make me among Your righteous servants.

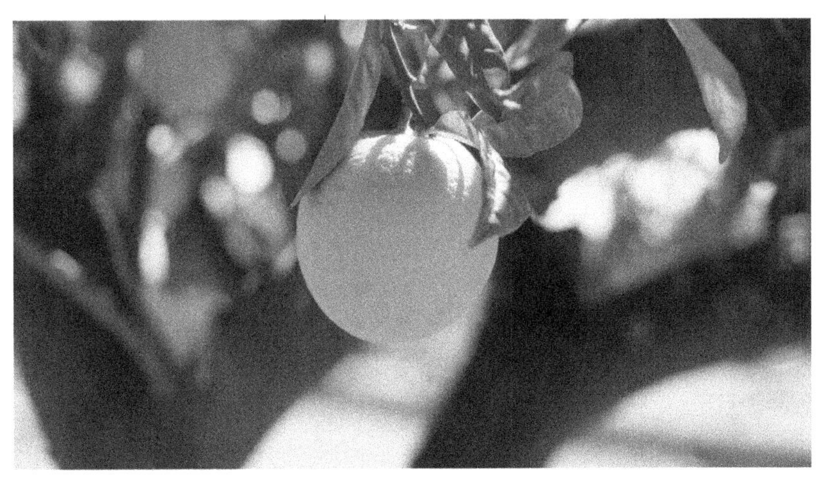

THE LAW OF **COMPOUNDING:** ITS DIVINE ORIGIN AND POTENTIAL FOR GOODNESS

The example of those who spend their wealth in the way of Allah is like a seed [of grain] which grows seven spikes; in each spike is a hundred grains. And Allah multiplies [His reward] for whom He wills. And

> *Allah is all-Encompassing and Knowing.* **Al-Quran 2:261**

In a world that demands more from us than we can handle, it's important to remember that doing the least is sometimes the most productive thing we can do. Don't burden yourself with excessive work, and don't let a fear of failure keep you from doing anything at all. Take comfort in the fact that even the smallest actions can have a tremendous impact. Imagine planting just one seed and how many people will ultimately benefit from the fruits it bears. From that one seed, countless trees could grow, feeding generations to come. The rewards of your small act could continue to multiply long after you're gone.

[Once upon a time, in the opulent court of a powerful monarch, there lived a humble peasant. The peasant, with his eyes filled with hope, approached the king with an unusual request. He asked the king for a mere grain of rice to be placed on a chessboard. Each day, the number of rice grains placed on it would be doubled and set on the next box, and so on, till the last block of the board. Initially the peasant's request seemed to be a trivial and harmless one but with each passing day, the number of rice grains on the chessboard multiplied at an astounding rate. By the time the chessboard reached its 19th block, it had already accumulated more than a million grains of rice and on the 64th block of the chessboard; there was not enough rice in the entire kingdom to satisfy the peasant's request.]

The law of compounding is a divine law that has been associated with interest (riba) by corrupt individuals. However, its original purpose was **not** to promote interest or to exponentially grow businesses, but rather to spread goodness and expand this world. The power of compounding is truly remarkable, as it has the potential to impact a massive number of people. Consider the fact that every human being who has ever lived in this world is a descendant of Adam and Eve, which amounts to billions of people. This is a testament to the immense power of the law of compounding.

Have You Heard of Sadaqa-e-Jarya: The Endless Impact of Compounding Deeds?This concept is a remarkable illustration of the compounding effect, where the goodness of one's actions continue to benefit countless people, long after their physical presence on earth. Sadaqa-e-Jarya, or ongoing charity, is an act of giving that creates an endless ripple of positive impact, impossible to count or measure.

How can we implement this law in our daily lives and in our communities?

One way to apply this law is by helping those in need, you don't have to solve the world hunger problem. Feed the nearest poor or help in education of a poor child. By doing so, you're not only helping them in the present, but you're also setting them up for a better future and potentially impacting their future generations as well. And the best part is, the effects of your actions keep compounding and multiplying even after you're gone. Even if you can help just a few people in your lifetime, you're already making a significant difference in the world.

Consider the power of compounding when it comes to good deeds and their impact on our **hereafter**. Did you know that despite there being only five daily prayers, you can still earn the reward of ten or more? Yes! By teaching someone to pray, and every time they perform their prayer, you'll also receive the reward. Similarly, there are only thirty days of fasting in Ramadan, but you can still earn the reward of sixty, a hundred, a thousand, or more days by providing iftar, **even if it's just a date**

[Take the first step]

> *Want to see the power of compounding in action? Try this experiment: grab your phone calculator and multiply 2x2. Then, hit the equal sign repeatedly and count how many clicks it takes to reach a million. The result will show you just how much impact even small actions can have when compounded over time.*

How Neglect Can Lead to Multiple Troubles ?

Unfortunately that the law of compounding is applicable to everything in our lives, including our problems. If you ignore a small issue, it is more likely to escalate into a bigger problem with time. To avoid such troubles, we must develop the habit of taking preventive measures.

For instance, if you have a cavity in one tooth and neglect it, it could affect the surrounding teeth as well. Similarly, if someone has diabetes and doesn't take necessary precautions, it can damage other organs in their body. Even something as simple as postponing your car maintenance could lead to costly repairs, medical bills, or even legal issues. Another example is a broken electric socket that you're putting off fixing. This minor issue could end up damaging your expensive electronic devices, and you may have to replace both the socket and the appliances.

Take small steps towards prevention, change the car tire as soon as it is due, and make sure to go for regular maintenance. Don't ignore a faulty electric socket, replace it as soon as you notice it. Don't delay going to the doctor for a regular check-up. One overlooked issue can lead to another and you might end up compounding the trouble. Remember, by doing the least you can save yourself from a lot of trouble.

The Power of Compounding in Learning

Have you ever noticed how knowing just one word in a foreign language can make it easier to learn related words and construct new sentences? Or how reading one book can open up a world of knowledge and lead to the discovery of many more books? The compounding effect of learning is remarkable - one small step can lead to a wealth of knowledge and understanding.

Compounding effect on Socializing.

How many direct friends you have, and how many friends' friends and relative you know. One acquaintance will lead to so many more.

The Compounding Effect on Social Connections: Have you ever thought about how knowing just one person can lead to knowing so many more? Consider the number of direct friends you have, and then think about their friends and relatives you know. One new acquaintance can expand your social circle exponentially

Business compounding effect:
As a business grows, its customer base increases gradually. Satisfying one customer will lead to another, and then another, and the compounding effect goes on and on

Instead of overwhelming yourself with unnecessary work, try to focus on doing the least amount of work that is necessary to achieve your goals. Working hard is not always the answer, sometimes working least can lead to better results

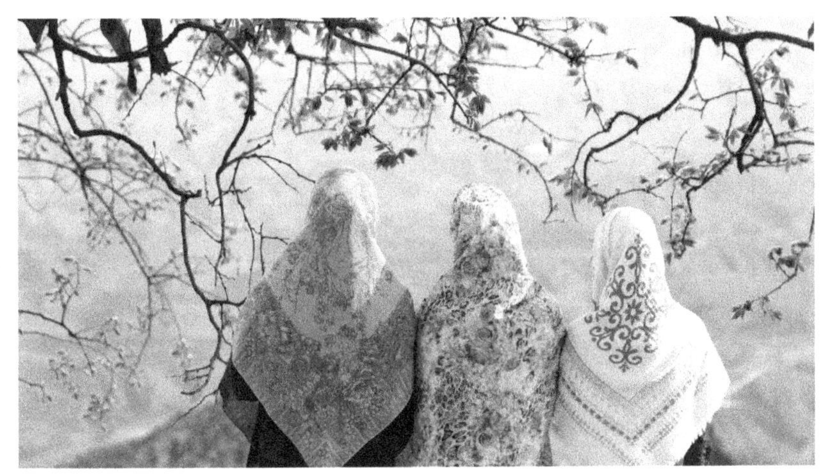

THE IMPORTANCE OF REAL **SOCIALIZING**: WHY TECHNOLOGY CAN'T REPLACE HUMAN CONNECTION

Do you ever truly feel fulfilled when socializing through a mobile screen? Social media technology may seem convenient, but it cannot replace the satisfaction of genuine human interaction. Instead, after an hour of mindless scrolling, we are often left feeling lonely, guilty, and envious. **Think about how much better it feels to spend time with good people,** time seems to fly. Yet, we often find ourselves consumed by daily soap operas on TV or Netflix series, lost in our own world. It's time to break free from these habits and seek out new connections. Make an effort to form new friendships and socialize in person. Studies show that people with friends tend to live longer and happier lives.

There's nothing that can alleviate worries faster than the reassurance of a friend saying "Insha'Allah, everything will be alright."

Friendship Knows No Age: Tips for Making Friends at Any Stage of Life

Making friends is not limited to just school years. It's possible to make friends at any point in our lives and it feels great to meet new people. Here are some tips for making new friends:

Find places where you can meet people who share similar interests as you.

Look for opportunities to strike up conversations with your neighbors, such as in the elevator, lobby, or parking area.

Visit different mosques or community centers to expand your social circle.

Take a leisurely stroll in the park instead of heading to a shopping mall.

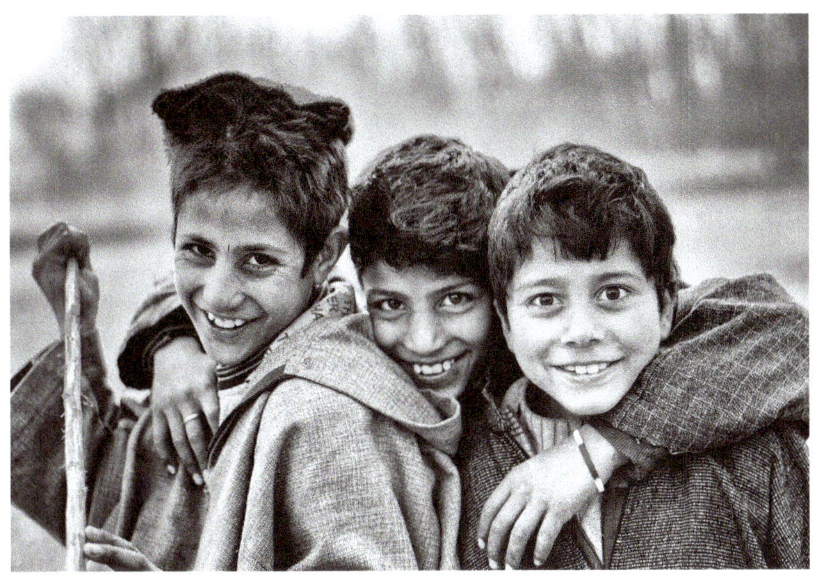

Ways for Introverted Muslims to Connect and Engage with Others.

Try these suggestions if you are not a social person and find it hard to enjoy being around people:

-Salam everyone. Host a small gathering at your home. *[A man asked the Messenger of Allah (PBUH): "Which act in Islam is the best?" He replied, "To give food, and to greet everyone, whether you know or you do not." Al-Bukhari and Muslim].*

-Smile often. *["Smiling in your brother's face is an act of charity" At-Tirmidhi "I have never seen anyone who smiles more than the Prophet does." At-Tirmidhi]*

-Look for opportunities to help others and be of service.

-Listen attentively and show sympathy to others to encourage and support them.

-Find ways to offer blessings (Dua) to everyone.

-Provide positive feedback to others.

-Make an effort to remember people's names, including your grocers, barber, mall checkout clerk, and others you interact with in your daily life. It can be fun to surprise someone by calling them by their name when they least expect it. Teaching your child to do the same can be a valuable lesson. Interestingly, people are often pleased to hear their name from a stranger or someone they do not anticipate to know them.

Create a regular schedule to meet up with friends or family. Choose a specific day of the week or month to visit or host a small gathering at home. Plan positive activities, such as studying the Quran, learning a new language, or reading together. Keep it short and sweet, avoiding lengthy and tedious events. When spending time with good company, disconnect from your phone and be present in the moment. Avoid giving the impression that you are disinterested or bored, such as through yawning.

The Company You Keep: Why It Matters

Human behavior is contagious. Research shows that we tend to mimic the behavior of those we spend the most time with. Have you ever noticed that when one person in a room yawns, it seems to trigger a chain reaction of yawns among others (did you just yawn)? It's a subconscious response that shows how easily we can be influenced by those around us.

Our earliest habits are not consciously chosen, but rather learned through imitation. The more we spend time with someone, the more likely we are to emulate their behavior. If you have ever found yourself in a foreign country or working in a diverse environment where people speak different languages or come from varying cultural backgrounds, you may have noticed yourself unconsciously adopting certain repetitive behaviors, small eating habits, or even their customary greetings, despite not knowing their language.

[Take the first step]
Challenge yourself to try something new. The next time you step out of your house, try to find someone's name and give them a friendly greeting. It's a small act of kindness that can brighten someone's day!

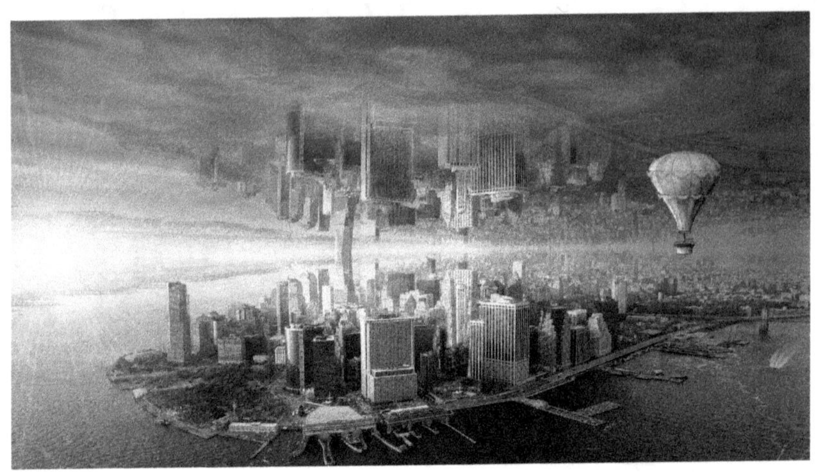

BELIEFS AND BEHAVIORS: THE POWER OF POSITIVE SELF-IMAGE

" OH ALLAH, MAKE ME EXTREMELY PATIENT, AND MAKE ME EXTREMELY GRATEFUL, AND MAKE ME INHERENTLY AND PERMANENTLY SMALL IN MY OWN EYES AND MAKE ME INHERENTLY AND PERMANENTLY GREAT IN THE EYES OF OTHERS "

[Take the first step]
Read this aloud "R E L A X"

Did you take a deep breath? It's interesting to note that your brain processes the words that you speak and your body reacts accordingly. Therefore, it's crucial to be mindful of the things you say about yourself, such as "I'm not good at this" or "I'm not that kind of person". When you hold the belief that you are a healthy and fit individual, you tend to prioritize your diet and exercise routine accordingly. Similarly, if you perceive yourself as a competent writer, you are more likely to put effort into enhancing your writing skills. Your actions are influenced by your beliefs, and the outcomes you desire will manifest as a result.

Changing your beliefs can change your identity. Here's an example - let's say two people want to cut down on sugar. When someone offers them a sugary drink, the first person might say, "No thanks, I'm trying to cut down on sugar." But the second person might say, "No thanks, I don't drink sugary beverages." It might seem like a small difference, but the language we use has a lot of power! The more we repeat a behavior, the more it becomes a part of our identity.

Repetition is key if you want to make a change stick!

You can't become a reader just by finishing one book or get fit after just one workout. Change takes time and happens gradually, day by day, little by little. It's only after consistently working out for a few months that you start to notice a change in your self-image. Every small step you take to improve your habits will eventually pay off. For example, every time you choose a no-sugar coffee, you're telling yourself that you care about your health and want to stay fit. The only way to change yourself is to change what you do. Unfortunately, this also applies to bad habits. Each time you engage in a bad habit, you're getting closer to that identity as well.

Build Self-Confidence with Positive *Affirmations* and Small Actions

It's important to give yourself a pat on the back every once in a while! If you just cleaned your room, take a moment to admire it and say to yourself "I like it clean." If you finished a page of a book, tell yourself "I like reading." When you're at a social gathering, remind yourself "I like being around good people." And if you just started reading the Quran, affirm to yourself "I love reading the Quran." However, remember that affirmation only works if you follow it up with action. It won't do any good to lay in bed after Fajr salah and say "I like to jog in the morning." You need to actually jog to convince yourself that you truly enjoy it.

Decide on the person you want to be and start proving it to yourself with small actions. Every small step you take towards becoming that person will make you more confident.

Want to help your kids feel even better about themselves? Try this out: Bring them some books that you think they might enjoy and say "Hey, I know you love reading, so I brought this book for you!" Whenever you see them doing something good, compliment them in a way that makes them feel like it's part of who they are, and try to get them to agree with you. For example, "Wow, you really like keeping your room clean, don't you?" or "You're always so helpful, aren't you?" Remember, it's important to avoid any negative feedback if possible!.

Use positive words when talking to yourself or your kids. Instead of saying "I am bad at this," say "I am a smart person and I will learn this quickly.

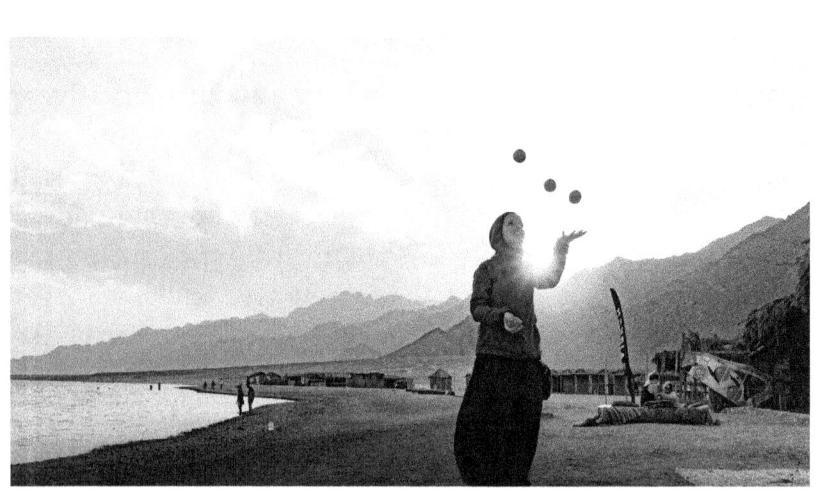

THE MYTH OF
MULTITASKING: HOW IT CAN
ACTUALLY SLOW YOU DOWN

Have you ever felt like there's just not enough time in a day to get everything done? It can be tough when we have high expectations for ourselves and feel like we're drowning in work. 24 hours are not enough for us anymore. We wish we could have more time in a day so that we could do more. You might think that multitasking is the answer, but it can actually slow us down as we switch between tasks and try to remember where we left off. Let's try to focus on one task at a time and give it our full attention. That way, we can be more efficient and get things done faster!

Why can't you do one thing at a time ?
In today's fast-paced world, it's easy to get caught up in the

idea of doing too many things at once. We often believe that multitasking is the key to getting more done in less time, but the truth is, it's just a myth. Our brains are not designed to handle multiple tasks at once like computers and smartphones, and trying to do so can actually slow us down. So the next time you're tempted to check your phone during dinner with your family, or talk to your kids while staring at a TV screen instead of looking at their eyes, or work on multiple projects simultaneously, remember that focusing on one thing at a time can actually be more productive in the long run. Take a deep breath, prioritize your tasks, and give your full attention to each one. You might just be surprised at how much more you can accomplish.

Do you still believe that multitasking is a productive way to get things done?

[Take the first step]
Let's try a simple experiment: try swinging one hand clockwise while moving the other hand up and down simultaneously.

Have you ever noticed how our minds are always on the go, either planning, worrying, or jumping from one task to another? This constant state of busyness is a result of our addiction to multitasking. We try to juggle multiple things at once, but in reality, it can have a negative impact on our mental health. For instance, while we work, we may be thinking about prayer, and while we pray, we may be thinking about the next task. Similarly, while doing chores, we may be distracted by social media status updates we are missing. All of this can lead to a sense of overwhelm and burnout.

I know what you might be thinking? That you could do some multitasking, like listening to the audiobook while taking a walk, driving, or doing daily chores. Your mind will still switch focus between three different things. Sometime your focus will be diverted to the job you are doing, and sometimes it goes wandering about the dreamland, or you start thinking about some un-finish job or some pressing problem. Only for a few minutes, you will come back to the audio.

Still not convinced? Try re-listening to the same chapter of the audiobook you were listening to while multitasking. You might realize that you missed good parts of it.

What is not a multitasking?

Reading a book while waiting for the doctor's appointment or listening to Quran while cooking are not multitasking because they don't require the same cognitive skills.

Breaking the habit of multitasking can be difficult, but it's essential to boost focus and improve performance. When you do one thing at a time with full attention, you'll finish tasks quicker and with greater accuracy.

If you're driving, avoid texting, as it requires the same cognitive skills. Similarly.
While studying, switch off the TV and keep your phone away to concentrate on the task at hand.
When you're with your friends or family, avoid checking your smartphone.
When your kids need attention, switch off the TV.

Focusing on one task at a time, you can become more productive.

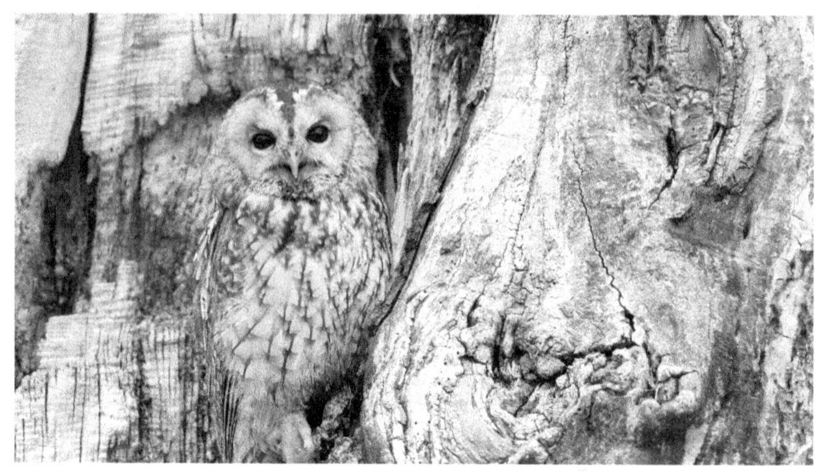

AVOID **DIGITAL DISTRACTIONS** : TAKE CONTROL OF YOUR FOUCS

The advent of smartphones has led to a decrease in human attention span, which is now shorter than that of a goldfish. However, we can still experience a state of mind called "focus," in which we are fully engaged in an activity and ***nothing else seems to matter***. This can be observed in athletes during competitions, people working on projects or meeting deadlines with only a few hours to spare.

Ask yourself, when was the last time you were in this state? Technology is constantly vying for our attention. Companies are pouring millions of dollars into getting and holding onto your focus. [**Focus** mispelled in title] It's crucial that we take action and recognize that attention is a valuable commodity. We've all experienced the constant stream of ads, recommendations, pop-ups, and mobile notifications that can feel overwhelming. [pay attention misspelled not *mispelled*]

Pomodoro

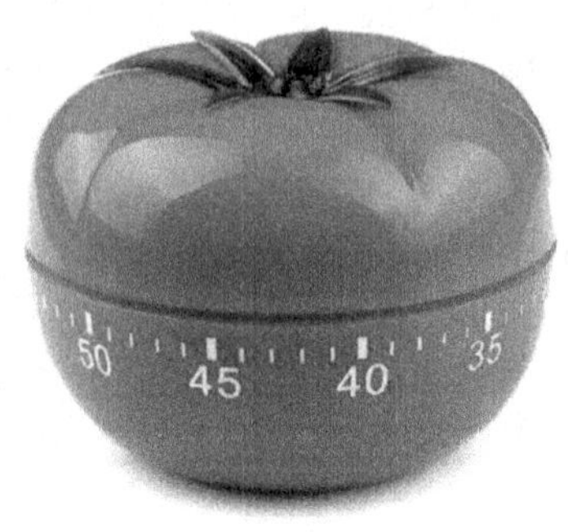

Have you heard of the Pomodoro study technique? It was invented by Francesco Cirillo and involves breaking tasks down into short timed intervals with breaks in between. All you need is a timer, but it's best to avoid using your smartphone's timer to minimize distractions.

Here's how it works:

- First, choose a task to work on.

- Set the timer for 20 minutes and focus on the task until the timer goes off (try not to keep checking the timer).

- When the timer goes off, take a short break for five minutes. It's important to move around and stretch your body, go to the bathroom, grab a glass of water, or do anything that helps you to relax.

- Avoid activities that could keep your mind engaged for longer than 5 minutes, such as checking social notifications. You could even meditate for 3 minutes if you want.

The main goal of the Pomodoro technique is to achieve an intense focus for 20 minutes. Our brains have limited attention spans, so we can only concentrate for a short time before getting distracted. Using a timer can help you to discipline yourself to focus on the task at hand by postponing any distractions until the break.While it may not work instantly, practicing this technique can lead to positive results. It's best to start with a smaller amount of work that is easier to get started on.

Do not confuse the 5-minute challenge with the Pomodoro technique. The 5-minute challenge is a method to get started and build momentum on a task, whereas the Pomodoro technique is designed for intense focus during a 20-minute cycle. If you're struggling to get started on a really boring task, you can begin with the 5-minute challenge to build some momentum. Once you feel like you're making progress, you can switch to the Pomodoro technique. These techniques are just tools to help you manage your time and attention more effectively. It's important to find what works best for you and adjust as needed.

When you need to focus on something, it's important to eliminate any potential distractions first. Consider putting your phone on airplane mode or keeping it in another room to avoid the temptation of constantly checking it. Even a brief distraction can disrupt your intense focus and lead your mind astray, making it difficult to get back on track. By removing potential distractions, you can increase your chances of staying focused and productive.

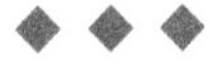

READ YOUR WAY
TO **RICHES**

Being rich isn't always about money or material possessions. It can also refer to having a wealth of knowledge, skills, **happiness**, or a rich heart. The irony is that a person who doesn't read often thinks they know everything, while a person who reads knows there is always more to learn. When you read, it's like downloading resources directly into your brain. You get to experience life through the perspective of someone else, and it can be truly eye-opening. For example, by reading 10 books by the age of 30, you could have the experience of 10 different people, each with their own unique perspective and insights to offer.

"Wealth is not in having many possessions. Rather,

> *true wealth is the richness of the soul." Ṣaḥīḥ al-*
> *Bukhārī 6081*

The person who reads and the person who doesn't read can't be the same. Nnowadays we have lots of resources to help you access information more easily than ever before. You can listen to book summaries, audiobooks, and there are even many great books available for free in the public domain. It's important to never stop learning, as studies have shown that reading can actually increase the size of your brain and expand your awareness.

Did you know that it's possible to learn a new skill within just 20 hours of dedicated practice? If you're skeptical, try committing to 20 hours of learning something new, such as coding, a foreign language, or even just memorizing the 400 most common words in a language. It's important to note that the 20 hours should be focused, deliberate practice, and not include time spent finding resources or making a plan. Give it a try and see the progress you can make in just 20 hours. It's amazing how much your understanding of the Quran can improve in just 20 hours! If you set a goal of dedicating 20 hours to learning and improving your Quranic Arabic, you can start by focusing on the most common 10 words in the Quran. Once you've mastered those, move on to learning the most common 100 words (at a pace of 5.5 words per hour, or approximately 10 minutes per word). To achieve this, you can set a target of learning 6 words per day for 20 days. In just 20 hours of focused study, you will be amazed at how much progress you can make. With the knowledge of the meanings and backgrounds of the Ayets, you will be able to understand more than 50% of the Quran, Insha'Allah.

How can I find an extra 10 minutes?

One way to save time on social media is to use an app that can block social media apps after a set amount of time. Alternatively, you could consider uninstalling all social media apps for a few days and only checking them once a day on your laptop.

Try a language learning experiment with your family. Find a list of the 400 most common words in any language and see how quickly you can learn and test your level after just 20 hours. Keep in mind that while this initial 20 hours can help you reach an intermediate level, it won't make you an expert in the skill. You can certainly learn the skill, but becoming an expert will take much more time and effort.

There is the rule of 10,000 hours, it says it takes 10k hours to become an expert in any skill, find it on the internet, it is very interesting. - (Seth Goldman 10,000 hours)

An initial 20 hours to learning a new skill can be a great way to spark interest and curiosity in children. This can help them discover a new passion or talent that they may want to pursue further. Additionally, this early success and boost in confidence can motivate them to continue practicing and developing their skills, potentially leading them to become experts in the field over time.

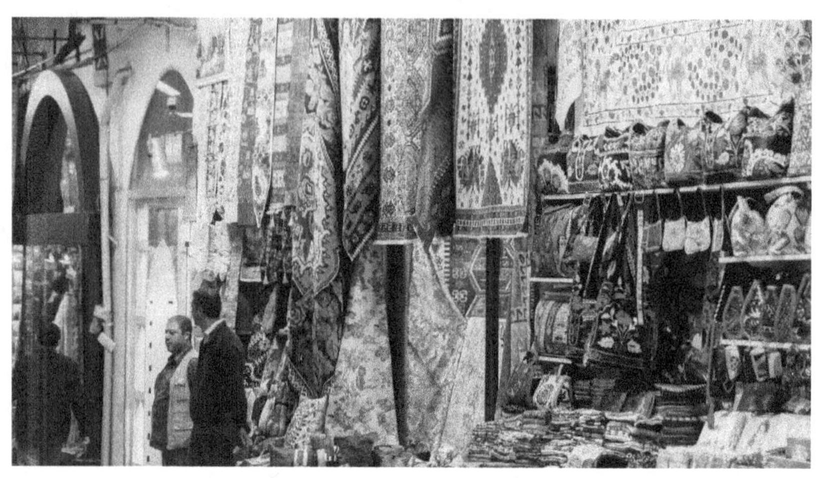

DON'T BUY A YOGA MAT : FINDING **PEACE** ON THE PRAYER MAT

AND WE SEND DOWN OF THE QUR'AN THAT WHICH IS
HEALING AND MERCY FOR THE BELIEVERS, BUT IT DOES
NOT INCREASE THE WRONGDOERS EXCEPT IN LOSS.
(QURAN: 17:82)

Have you ever heard of the prayer mat called Sajjada that Muslims use for their five daily prayers? Well, you can actually use it for meditation too! Did you know that Salah, which is the Islamic form of prayer, is similar to yoga but with even greater benefits? And guess what, reciting the Quran can be incredibly powerful for your well-being. It has been known to release fears, anxiety, and guilt, while also reducing blood pressure and stress levels. Give it a try and see how it brings you **peace**.

[Take the first step]
Monitor your breath the moment you start reading or listening to the Quran.

If you're ever feeling stressed or worried, here's a tip: try praying two extra Rakat. It's a great way to calm your mind and ease anxiety. When you disconnect from the world and connect with Allah, you can leave your worries on Sajjada and feel a sense of **peace**. And if your worries start to creep back in during Salah, just remind yourself that you're standing in front of the Almighty, who created and runs this world. To really focus on your prayer, take a quick 10-minute break from everything else beforehand.

-Make sure to turn off the stove and don't leave anything on the burner, so your mind doesn't keep taking you back to the kitchen.

-Put your mobile on silent mode, or consider using driving mode to let callers know you'll call them back when it's convenient. Unless it's an emergency, they can wait.
-Keep your prayer area clean and free of clutter, as a cluttered space can distract your mind and cause you to forget about your Salah.

-Choose a simple Sajjada (prayer mat) design. Intricate patterns or designs may attract your attention and distract your mind, taking away from your prayerful focus.

-One of the best ways to improve your Salah experience is by preparing yourself before it's time to pray. Make it a habit to spread out your Sajjada and sit in readiness for Salah at least 3 minutes before it begins. This can be a rewarding practice that allows you to disconnect from the things that were previously occupying your mind. Remember, it takes time for your mind to shift its focus from one activity to another. By giving yourself this brief window of time to prepare, you'll be better able to fully immerse yourself in your prayer and get the most out of your Salah.

[Take the first step]
Listen to Qural on YouTube and monitor your body's response. You might be surprised to find that you take a deep breath and your body begins to relax almost instantly.

Listening to Quranic recitation can be a powerful tool for reducing stress and promoting a sense of calm. Give it a try next time you're feeling overwhelmed - you just might find it helps you feel more centered and relaxed.

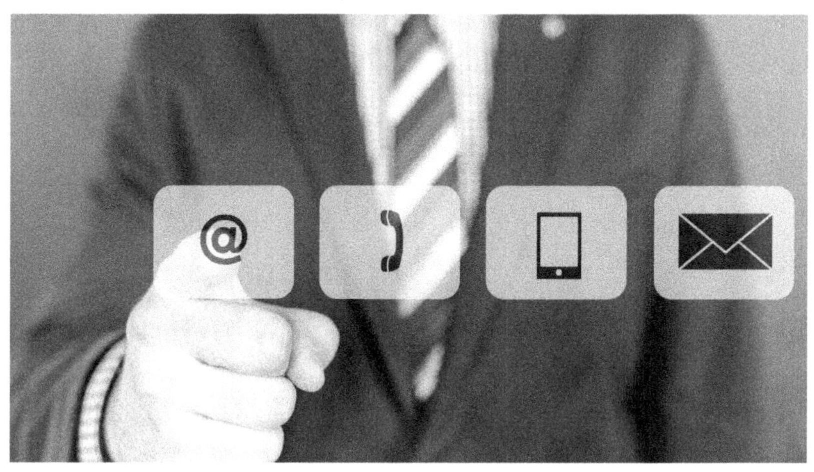

CONNECT WITH US

nue**worth**@gmail.com

Thank you for taking the time to read my book. I hope you found it useful and it met your expectations. If you have any comments, feedback, or suggestions, please do not hesitate to contact me. It will help me improve my next edition.

Remember me in your prayers and if you enjoyed reading the book, please leave a review . Your review can help others make an informed decision about whether to read this book or not.